Casemix for All

EDITED BY

HUGH SANDERSON
PHIL ANTHONY

AND

LEONIE MOUNTNEY

FOREWORD BY

PETER LEES

RADCLIFFE MEDICAL PRESS

© 1998 Hugh Sanderson, Phil Anthony and Leonie Mountney

Radcliffe Medical Press Ltd
18 Marcham Road, Abingdon, Oxon OX14 1AA, UK

British Library Cataloguing in Publication Data

A catalogue record for this book is available from the British Library.

ISBN 1 85775 217 1

Library of Congress Cataloging-in-Publication Data is available.

Typeset by Advance Typesetting Ltd, Oxfordshire
Printed and bound by Biddles Ltd, Guildford and King's Lynn

Contents

Foreword

As the tension between the provision, rising demand and cost of health care achieves increasing national prominence, it is especially important that meaningful measures of health care are developed which define need and accurately quantify resource consumption.

Casemix is the science of classifying and quantifying the use of health care resources and, in England and Scotland, Healthcare Resource Groups (HRGs) are the measurement tool. Healthcare Resource Groups define resource use on the basis of the treatment profile to produce a multi-purpose set of groupings which are usable and understood by clinicians and managers. Interestingly, by combining clinical and resource data, groupings often have different, but highly relevant meanings for clinicians and managers and can be a useful language to facilitate dialogue between the two groups.

Casemix is not a new concept, its roots originating in the USA in the 1970s. Healthcare Resource Groups, the English equivalent of the 'parent' US system – Diagnosis Related Groups – were developed in response to the Resource Management Initiative in 1986, and were given greater impetus by the introduction of the Internal Market to the National Health Service (NHS). The latest White Paper, *The New NHS* (December 1997) has increased the focus on performance management of efficiency and effectiveness and HRGs will provide the basis for benchmarking activity costs. Consequently, HRGs are now in widespread use in the UK, and will shortly be mandatory in all specialties for costing and pricing. From this flows their use for agreement specification and monitoring, service planning and national comparisons, and these functions will be enhanced by their combination with Health Benefit Groups (HBGs) as a way of categorizing the need in the population.

The success and value of HRGs in the UK can be directly credited to the editors of this book. Hugh Sanderson, Phil Anthony and Leonie Mountney have led the development and implementation of casemix for the NHS through the National Casemix Office and its network, including the clinician-led specialty working groups. The network is reflected in the diverse range of contributors to this book, who include the recognized theoretical experts in the casemix field and a wide range of practical users from primary and secondary care, and from finance, contracting and clinical staff.

Casemix for All covers present and future topics, and touches on the more difficult areas of mental health and community and primary care. It also includes valuable case studies drawn from expert users. The resulting blend gives the book a broad appeal to those in the front line of managing clinical services, who cannot afford to be ignorant of casemix, its use and its implications.

PETER LEES
Chairman, British Association of Medical Managers
Consultant Neurosurgeon and Director of Research,
Southampton University Hospitals NHS Trust
January 1998

With grateful thanks to Bob Logan, Emeritus Professor of Medical Care, London School of Hygiene and Tropical Medicine, who created the opportunity and provided the encouragement for the start of casemix studies in this country; and to Tim Scott, who ensured their continuation through the Resource Management Programme.

Preface

ANYONE working in the NHS who has some responsibility for the management of the delivery of services to patients needs to have information about the types of patients they are serving, the types of care provided and the results that they have achieved. This has of course always been true, but the increasing costs and demands on the NHS and the increasing availability of information makes it even more important for managers to be able to use this information effectively.

Casemix for All helps the reader to a better understanding of the principles and purposes of casemix and explains the way in which these concepts have been turned into practical casemix groupings, both in this and other countries. It also provides the reader with some practical examples of how the application of casemix groupings to patient data has helped to improve the management of services.

The book also highlights the enormous potential of casemix analysis, not only now, but also in the future, when clinical systems will provide highly detailed and accurate clinical information for statistical analysis. There is much under-exploited potential that can be used now, but we should realize that a future potential also exists, and be aware that when clinical systems are widely available, we will be able to use the data within them for very useful purposes.

The concept of casemix is therefore at a cross-roads: the methods that are available now need to be exploited, and also the future methods of grouping data need to be considered. These will alter radically the ways in which we think about casemix, the development of data systems and the ways in which data can be analysed to improve the management of health services.

Casemix for All should be read by health service managers and clinicians who have some management responsibilities within the NHS, whether they are in a purchaser or in a provider organization, in primary, community or secondary hospital care settings. In particular, it focuses on the difference between groupings of patients with conditions and groupings of intervention episodes and the way in which these two separate types of groupings can be used in isolation and together to improve understanding of the performance of health services. This is not just for the acute services (which has been the traditional domain of casemix groups), but as a way of understanding the complete spectrum of services required for a wide range of conditions, from individuals who are at risk, to those with irreversible and progressive disease.

It also discusses the application of these casemix grouping methods to particular health service management problems and includes chapters from contributors who have been using casemix groupings as purchasers (both at health authority and general practitioner (GP) level), as providers and also within provider organizations.

Chapter 5, by Rod Smith, David Archer and Fran Butler identifies issues in the use of HRGs from a GP purchasing perspective, and the ways in which cost information and clinical performance can be assessed. Chapter 6, by Alan Butler, Jeremy Horgan and Lisa Macfarlane from Southampton University Hospitals Trust shows how HRGs have been used to support the development of clinical directorates and the negotiation of contracts with purchasers. Chapter 7, also from a provider perspective by Nigel Woodcock and Ken Lloyd from Northampton, identifies how HRGs have been used to examine quality of care, and to support service developments. Chapter 8, by David Meechan discusses how HRGs have been used to support and monitor contracts by Doncaster Health Authority. Chapter 9, by Tim Scott discusses the use of casemix groups by clinical directors for the purpose of managing their clinical directorates.

These contributions are focused mainly on the use of groupings of treatment episodes, HRGs, since these are more widely available at present. Chapter 10, however, by Andrew Walker from the Greater Glasgow Health Board and colleagues discusses the pilot experience of using both condition-based groups (Health Benefit Groups (HBGs)) and treatment episodes (HRGs). In particular it describes the difficulties of obtaining the data at present, and the potential applications for commissioning and monitoring the services required to meet the needs of the population.

Casemix for All is not intended to be a manual of how to use the grouping software (whether for HRGs, Diagnosis Related Groups (DRGs), Disease Staging or some other grouping method), nor a manual for describing how to process records that have been allocated into groups. It is, however, a book which explains why casemix groups are useful and the reasons for grouping and analysing patient records.

The structure and application of casemix groupings is very dependent on the health care system, and particularly the method of funding in existence. For this reason, the way in which grouping systems are used varies between countries. Since health care systems are developing constantly, it follows that the application and design of grouping systems need to change and adapt, and for this reason the work of developing patient groupings is dynamic. There is much work still to be done in exploring the concepts, developing new and better groupings of patients and health care activities and applying them to improve the management of health services. This book raises some of the unresolved issues and points to potential developments that may deal with current problems. Since it is also true that some of the recent developments in health care systems are dependent upon (and may even be driven by) the improved availability of information, consideration is given to how developments in the construction of casemix groupings could be used to develop equitable and effective health services.

The book has been written at a time when the White Paper, *The New NHS*, will emphasize the use of casemix in the NHS. However, whatever structure of organization and allocation of resources is employed in any health care system, it is likely that ways of identifying the needs and costs of care will be important. We anticipate that much of the material contained in this book will become increasingly relevant, both in the UK and elsewhere.

Many colleagues within the NHS, the NHS Executive and in other countries have contributed to the development of our ideas and knowledge. Particular thanks go to all of the members of the National Casemix Office who have participated in many of the internal discussions, to the members of the clinical working groups and project boards who have helped and guided the development of casemix in England, and to those colleagues within the Patient Classification Systems in Europe (PCSE) association, who have helped us to see the issues within the NHS from an international perspective.

Finally, our thanks are due to Lesley Morris for her long-suffering patience in typing and administrative support.

HUGH SANDERSON, PHIL ANTHONY AND LEONIE MOUNTNEY
January 1998

List of contributors

David Archer
General Practitioner
Lincoln House Surgery
Wolsey Road
Hemel Hempstead
Herts HP2 4SH

Harry Burns
Director of Public Health
Greater Glasgow Health
  Board
Dalian House
350 St Vincent Street
Glasgow G3 8YU

Alan Butler
Director of Finance and
  Information
Southampton University Hospitals
  Trust
Tremona Road
Southampton SO16 6YD

Fran Butler
Project Manager
Berkshire Integrated Purchasing
  Project
Berkshire Health Authority
57–59 Bath Road
Reading
Berks RG30 2BA

Jeremy Horgan
Costing Development
  Manager
Healthcare Analysis Research
  Unit
Southampton University Hospitals
  Trust
Tremona Road
Southampton SO16 6YD

Karen Jack
Research Assistant
Accounts Commission for
  Scotland
18 George Street
Edinburgh EH2 2QU

Ken Lloyd
Former Chief Executive
Northampton General
  Hospital
Billing Road
Northampton NN1 5BD

Lisa Macfarlane
Healthcare Analysis Research
  Unit
Southampton University Hospitals
  Trust
Tremona Road
Southampton SO16 6YD

David Meechan
Director of Research and
    Information
Doncaster Health Authority
White Rose House
Ten Pound Walk
Doncaster DN4 5DJ

Leonie Mountney
Operational Director
National Casemix Office
Highcroft
Romsey Road
Winchester
Hants SO22 5DH

Hugh Sanderson
Director
National Casemix Office
Highcroft
Romsey Road
Winchester
Hants SO22 5DH

Tim Scott
Senior Fellow
BAMM
Barnes Hospital
Cheadle
Cheshire SK8 2NY

Rod Smith
General Practitioner
Balmore Park Surgery
59a Hemdean Road
Caversham
Berks RG4 7SS

Sara Twaddle
Director of Research and
    Audit
Stobhill Hospital NHS
    Trust
Balomock Road
Glasgow G21 3UW

Andrew Walker
Greater Glasgow Health
    Board
Dalian House
350 St Vincent Street
Glasgow G3 8YU

Nigel Woodcock
Deputy Chief Executive/Director
    of Finance
Northampton General
    Hospital
Billing Road
Northampton NN1 5BD

1   The philosophy and concepts
       of casemix

Classification and grouping

Classification of events in the outside world is fundamental to organizing knowledge. In order to survive, our ancestors in the hunter/gatherer stage of evolutionary history needed to classify animals into those they could eat and those that could eat them. Such a simple classification inevitably becomes more complex; perhaps subdividing into those animals that were really good to eat, those that were not so good, and those which could be eaten if there was nothing else. Similarly, there were animals who were very likely to eat our ancestors, which they needed to keep well away from, and those animals which ate humans only under extreme circumstances and which they could ignore for most of the time.

In exactly the same way, in describing patients and activities in health services, we need to be able to classify those patients and the activities provided to patients, in order to describe them and predict their needs for care or the prognosis of treatment. Of course, since every individual is unique, every patient is unique and every treatment is unique, but at some level of generalization it is possible to identify the common characteristics of patients and the common characteristics of their treatments. Indeed, without such an ability to classify, there would be no knowledge, there would be no medical or nursing textbooks and there would be no clinical trials or evidence-based medicine. Classification of patients has been undertaken for many years. One of the early examples of the uses of classification for statistical reporting was the *London Bills of Mortality*, by John Graunt,[1] developed in the 17th Century. Over time, these systems developed into the International Classification of Diseases (ICD),[2] which has been widely adopted across the world for the purpose of reporting mortality and morbidity.

All classifications however are a balance between precision and practicality and the level of detail within a classification is dependent on its purpose. To an entomologist there are several million species of insects and the distinction between each species is important. To a lay person there may be 20 or 30 important types of insect, and the rest are bugs, creepy-crawlies, flies or just 'insects'. The level of detail may also depend on the focus of interest. Gardeners will know about insects that damage vegetables and fruits (such as aphids, red spider mites, codling moths, cabbage-white butterflies, etc.), fishermen may be interested in insects that are eaten by fish (mayflies, caddis flies, etc.), householders may be interested in wood-eating insects (woodworm, death-watch beetle, etc.). So it is with health care. For some purposes it may be sufficient to know whether a patient has cardiovascular disease or musculoskeletal disease, but for other purposes whether the patient has a posterior or an anterior myocardial infarct is of great importance and significance. Some clinicians will want to know about endocrine disorders in great detail, but this may be of little interest to others who want to know a great deal about respiratory disease.

Casemix grouping is the grouping together of similar conditions or interventions for various analytical purposes, and so the work of developing casemix groups depends upon achieving an appropriate compromise between the level of specificity and their purpose. For example, the purpose may be to understand the costs of care at a general hospital level, and in that instance the groupings might be less detailed than the groupings developed to identify the costs of highly complex cases within a regional or national specialty. These groupings would however be quite different from the groups developed to predict the outcome of care for particular conditions; in this instance the classification would be organized around the characteristics of patients' conditions which predict good or bad outcomes. For the former purpose, the classification would be organized around the characteristics of treatment episodes which predict high or low cost.

For the purpose of analysis in the sort of groupings that are in general labelled as casemix, the intention is to describe the work of a hospital or other clinical unit in a manageable number of groups (perhaps ten to 20 for a particular clinical department). But this is not the only level at which analysis may be useful, and for clinical management purposes, these groups may need to be broken down into more precise types of patients or interventions.

In general, classification is the same process as grouping, and vice versa. Groupings and classifications may be multi-axial (based upon several different variables), and they may also have several levels of aggregation. However, in common parlance, casemix groupings exist somewhere between the level of specialty or department and those classifications, such as the ICD, or procedure code classifications (e.g. Office of Population Census and Surveys (OPCS) procedure codes,[3] etc.). These have thousands of classes within them – ICD 10 has more than 10 000, OPCS 4 has more than 6000.

At a more discrete level are terming/nomenclature systems, such as Read Codes[4] or the Systematised Nomenclature of Medicine (SNOMED),[5] which

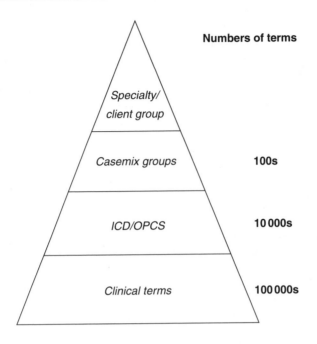

Figure 1.1: The 'language of health' pyramid.

may have tens- or hundreds of thousands of classes. The common purpose of these groupings or classifications is to enable comparisons and predictions, and the precision of the grouping required depends upon the purpose of the comparison. This arrangement is very similar to an Executive Information Pyramid in which the level of aggregation of information is related to the level of decision making required. This concept has been labelled as the Language of Health (see Figure 1.1), in which a common theme of a language holds the elements of terms, classifications and groupings together. Similar to the languages used to communicate between people, the Language of Health has a purpose in enabling communication, but requires a common understanding of the building blocks (the words, or clinical terms) and an agreed way of putting those words together to communicate more complex meanings. In a similar way, the combination and aggregation of terms into classifications and groups function to enable the communication of more complex concepts.[6]

That the grouping of cases is a fundamental step in analysis of data seems to be obvious. What may not be so obvious however, is the reason for having grouping systems set up as national or international standards. The reasons are two-fold. The first is in terms of efficiency, since the underlying coding systems are complex it would be costly and wasteful to have highly skilled individuals specifying groupings and writing software in each place that wanted to analyse patient data. (In addition, there are not enough analysts with the skills available in the NHS.) The second reason is to enable comparability, since only if the groupings used in one place are similar to another can informed comparisons be made. Using standard groupings enables benchmarking and comparisons of the efficiency and effectiveness of one locality against others.

Groupings of conditions and interventions

Within any health care system a very simple model of care delivery can be applied which provides a useful way to understand the development and uses of casemix. This model (adapted from Iezzoni[7]) identifies a patient (with an actual or potential condition) receiving an activity (prevention/assessment/treatment/care, etc.) which results in an outcome.

Patient + Intervention = Outcome

This very simplified relationship provides two key axes for the grouping of patient information. These are the axes of patient conditions and of health service activity.

Different conditions of course, require different interventions, and as a general rule the condition/intervention relationship encompasses all conditions and health service activities.

Table 1.1 shows that, at each stage (from being at-risk to irreversible disease), there are different objectives of care, and the location of care primarily takes place in different services.

This general model works reasonably well to describe the components of health care, and the way in which they are deployed to meet the needs of the population. However, it is important to recognize that the classification of conditions is different at different stages of the process. For example, individuals at-risk can be classified in terms of behaviours (smokers, those who are overweight, etc.) or genetic risk (for example, family history of breast cancer). Those with symptoms are described in terms of the symptoms they report, but those with reversible disease will be classified in terms of pathology (coronary artery disease, lung cancer, etc.), whilst those with irreversible disease may be classified in terms of their functional abilities (mobility, activities of daily living, etc.). These different dimensions of conditions are related to the interventions required, and there are important differences in the language and philosophy of care in different health care

Table 1.1:   Conditions, interventions and objectives

Type of condition	Type of intervention	Objective	Health care sector
At low risk (normal population)	Promotion	Reduce risk	Community/primary care
At specific risk	Prevention	Prevent disease	Community/primary care
Symptoms	Diagnostic tests/assessment	Confirm/exclude diagnosis	Primary/outpatient/ day care
Reversible disease	Treatment	Cure	Primary/outpatient/ inpatient care
Irreversible disease	Care/support/ pain relief	Care	Primary/community/ long-stay care

sectors, because they have quite different objectives for the care provided. These differences are particularly marked between the acute and community sectors, and since much of the development of casemix groups has taken place in the acute sector, there can be a tendency for community services to reject the casemix approach as being inappropriate. From this general perspective, this is clearly not the case, but the groupings of conditions and interventions need to be defined in appropriate terms. The same issues apply to social care, again, the general model of conditions and interventions can apply, but the language and organization of services are different, and groupings may need to be defined in different ways.

The purpose of casemix groups

If casemix groups are used to identify types of patients and types of activity, then whether the activity provided is appropriate for that condition can be established. Whether the activity is being provided as efficiently as possible and if the outcome of that treatment for that condition was as good and as effective as expected can also be established.

Appropriateness, efficiency and effectiveness are fundamental dimensions to the delivery of a cost-effective service and there is considerable evidence that there is variation between places in all of these dimensions. By enabling comparisons, managers and clinicians can identify how to perform better, and provide a more cost-effective service for their community.

In addition, understanding of the rates of interventions in relation to the prevalence of a condition is very important in assessing the equity of access to care. There is a large volume of literature on the variations in utilization rates for particular conditions which has frequently suggested that differences in incidence or prevalence are much less important than variations in medical practice or the availability of resources.[8] These sources of inequity of access can also be addressed by using patient-based data, grouped into casemix groups for comparisons.

The condition/intervention group matrix

A convenient and easy to visualize way of combining the two axes is to set out condition and intervention groups as a two-dimensional matrix (Table 1.2). In this way it is possible to identify the intervention group appropriate for a particular condition group.

Table 1.2: The condition/intervention group matrix

Conditions	Interventions			
	HRG 1	HRG 2	HRG 3	etc
Health Benefit Group (HBG) A		X		
HBG B	X		X	
HBG C			X	
etc				

This is a very simplified model, but can be used to demonstrate a number of fundamental points.

- In some instances a single intervention is appropriate for a particular type of condition and provides all the care required for that episode of illness. For example, appendicectomy for acute appendicitis.
- In other instances, more than one treatment process may be required for a single condition. This might be because immediate and longer term care are required, or it may be that there are options for the most appropriate treatment package for a particular condition.
- There is a possibility that a particular intervention may be appropriate for more than one condition, for example the rehabilitation package provided both for patients with head injury and those with stroke.

This model needs to be made more complex to deal with a wide range of types of conditions and interventions, but in principle the matrix can be constructed to show each of the types of condition and relevant intervention. Table 1.3 shows the general structure (with the objective of care in the relevant section as identified in Table 1.1).

Table 1.3: General structure

	Promotion/ prevention	Diagnostic/ assessment	Curative	Caring/ supporting
At-risk	Reduce risk, prevent disease			
Symptoms		Confirm/exclude diagnosis		
Reversible disease			Cure	
Irreversible disease				Care, support, palliation

Representing this as four separate, but linked matrices, for cancer of the breast as shown in outline in the Appendix on p. 9 demonstrates the processes of care for the whole course of the condition from at-risk to widespread irreversible disease. This includes activities in primary care, outpatient settings, inpatients, and hospital- or community-based palliative care.

This approach for cancer of the breast could be used to help decide the packages of care that should be delivered to meet the defined population needs for these individuals, and by aggregation to identify the resources that might be required in terms of facilities, equipment, staffing and expertise. Since the provision of resources often owes more to history than to rational allocation, it may well be that there is a mismatch between the resources and activity expected, and that delivered.

Services could also be monitored in this way. The matrix permits the specification of standards of structure and process for the delivery of each intervention package (these might be in several areas, including standards of training and qualification of staff, service standards for patients, and measures of access and equity), as well as identifying the expected outcomes of care for each condition group. In the Appendix example outcome measures are shown in the righthand column, and the process indicators in the bottom rows of the matrix. In addition, both the cost expected for the service can be compared with the actual cost, and the outcomes expected compared with those achieved. The indicators in the Appendix are examples only but are used to demonstrate the potential use of groupings to integrate the information required both to plan and monitor the delivery of health care.

In simple terms, condition groups may be seen as of primary interest to purchasers since they describe the epidemiology of the population. Intervention groups are of more interest to providers since they can describe the cost of delivering a particular intervention. However, using a combination of groupings of conditions and interventions has potential for managing the whole health care system from a population-based perspective, and enabling a constructive dialogue between purchaser and provider.

Practical issues in developing a matrix of condition and intervention groups

The separation into groups of conditions and interventions is not a new idea,[9] but it does help to clarify the characteristics of the various grouping schemes that have been developed, and helps to identify their value for various different purposes. There are however a number of issues that need to be addressed in moving from the theory to the practical construction and use of these groups. These issues revolve about the definitions and capture of data, and are discussed in more detail in Chapters 2 and 3.

A more detailed discussion of the practical issues surrounding the application of casemix methods is provided in the case studies in Chapters 6 to 10. These focus mainly on the use of groups of interventions in acute inpatient care (inpatient Healthcare Resource Groups), since these are the only ones available at the present time.

References

1   Greenwood M (1948) *Medical Statistics from Graunt to Farr*. Cambridge University Press, Cambridge.
2   World Health Organisation (1994) *International Classification of Diseases*. 10th revision. WHO, Geneva.
3   Office of Population Census and Surveys (1990) *Classification of Surgical Operations and Procedures*. 4th revision. HMSO, London.
4   Chisholm J (1990) The Read Clinical Classification. *BMJ* **300**: 1092.
5   Cote RA (ed.) (1993) *Systematised Nomenclature of Medicine (SNOMED) International*. College of American Pathologists, Chicago.
6   Read JD, Sanderson HF and Drennan YM (1995) Terming , Encoding and Grouping. *Medinfo 95 Proceedings* **1**: 56–9.
7   Iezzoni LI, Ash AS, Coffman GA *et al.* (1992) Predicting In-Hospital Mortality: A Comparison of Severity Measurement Approaches. *Medical Care* **30**: 347–59.
8   Wennberg JE, Freeman JL and Culp WJ (1987) Are Hospital Services Rationed in Newhaven or Overutilised in Boston? *Lancet* **i**: 1185–9.
9   Hornbrook MC (1982) Hospital case mix: its definition, measurement and use. Part I. The conceptual framework. *Medical Care Review* **39**: 1–43.

Appendix: Breast cancer HBG/HRG matrix

Health outcome indicators are given in the righthand column (shaded) and process indicators are given in the bottom rows (shaded).

HBGs →	HRGs →	Promotion	Prevention	Diagnostic/ Assessment	Cure	Caring/ Supporting	Health outcome indicators	
							Technical	Consumer
HBGs →		Reduce exposed population	Reduce progression to disease	Confirm/exclude diagnosis	Return to health/ reduce avoidable complications	Improve quality of life/ reduce avoidable complications		
At-risk I	Whole female population	Health promotion						Acceptability of health promotion
At-risk II	Population at specific risk\n\nPrevious breast cancer		Breast awareness Mammography Prophylactic mastectomy				Rate of early detection	Acceptability of screening
Symptoms	Asymptomatic, mammogram +ve\n\nSymptomatic			Mammogram/ ultrasound/chest X-ray/fine-needle aspiration/excision biopsy/skeletal survey			Sensitivity/ Specificity	Satisfied with diagnostic testing

Appendix: Continued

HRGs →	Promotion	Prevention	Diagnostic/Assessment	Cure	Caring/Supporting	Health outcome indicators	
						Technical	Consumer
Reversible disease	Non-invasive breast cancer Early stage Locally advanced Metastatic				Surgery/ chemotherapy/ radiotherapy/ special support		Survival rates by stage	Patient satisfaction
Irreversible disease	Disability Pain					Community/ specialist/ palliative care		Patient/ relative satisfaction
Process indicators: appropriateness			Coverage of breast cancer screening	Percentage with one-stop diagnosis	Standardized treatment rates by type, e.g. surgery	Provision of terminal care		
Equity			Percentage eligible females screened		Percentage with appropriate treatment	Percentage with accredited palliative care		
Efficiency		Cost	Cost/early breast cancer detected	Cost/diagnosed breast cancer	Cost/curative treatment course	Cost/care course		
Cost		££	££	££	££	££		

2   Resource groupings: history of development and current state

THE discussion in Chapter 1 referred to the potential for describing conditions and interventions in a four-stage process, based upon the objectives of care and including measures of process and outcome quality. This functional classification of interventions does not fit exactly to the organizational classification of health care (primary, secondary [inpatient/outpatient] and tertiary care) which is more commonly used to describe health care services, but in practice, most preventive/promotion care is provided in primary care, and most of inpatient hospital care is curative (although there is a substantial amount of caring service also). Diagnostic/assessment services may be primary- or secondary-care based, and within the secondary care setting may be inpatient or outpatient. Despite this overlap between some categories, it is worth persisting with a casemix resource grouping classification based on the objective of care, because when planning the services required it may be more important to identify *what* the need is rather than *where* the service is provided. Indeed, the changing structures of health services enable the delivery of health care in many different settings, and the development of policies around the concepts of 'seamless care' means that the distinctions between primary and secondary care are increasingly blurred and unhelpful.

Much of the work on casemix has however been done on acute inpatient episodes, since this is where the data are available, and where the majority of the costs are incurred, and inevitably this area will receive the main focus in this chapter. However, it is important to remember that these issues also relate in greater or lesser ways to the grouping of patient episodes for the purposes of prevention, diagnostic assessment, care and support.

Inpatient groupings

As in many other countries, the NHS in England collects a patient-based set of information about hospital activity. This was initiated with a 10% sample return in the 1950s (the Hospital Inpatient Enquiry (HIPE)),[1] and developed into full-scale hospital data sets collected at a regional level in the 1970s (Hospital Activity Analysis),[2] which were eventually consolidated into the Korner Hospital Episodes Statistics (HES) returned to the Department of Health since 1986.

Similar processes have occurred in other European countries with the development and endorsement by the EU of a Minimum Basic Data Set,[3] and within the USA, with the development of a Uniform Hospital Abstract, which has emerged as a Minimum Basic Data Set. These data sets have in general used the ICD to capture diagnostic information (although the USA has used a clinical modification (ICD9-CM) for the last 15 years), but there has been less standardization of the classification of surgical procedures. Most countries have, until fairly recently, developed and used their own system of surgical procedure classification. Only in the last ten years has the procedure classification within the ICD9-CM scheme, developed in the USA, become more widely adopted. In the UK, the OPCS started the development of a procedure classification for use in HIPE in the 1950s, this has been updated over the years, and the current version, OPCS4,[4] was implemented in 1988.

These classifications of diseases and procedures have been used for statistical reporting and, as a result, short-lists of codes, either using chapter headings or aggregations of particular conditions, have been available for a number of years (e.g. The Basic Tabulation list and the Mortality list within ICD 9). In the 1970s however interest, particularly in the USA, turned towards trying to classify the outputs, or products, of hospitals in a more systematic and statistically driven way.

Criteria for resource groups

The criteria used in the development of these classifications of episodes of care (hospital products/outputs) have been summarized by Fetter and his colleagues[5] who identified four key characteristics to be included in the design, and these have been generally accepted as the model for subsequent developments.

1 The episodes within any one group should be similar in their expected use of resources.
2 The episodes within each group should be clinically similar, and involve reasonably similar processes.
3 Allocation of cases into a group should be on the basis of variables within the routinely collected minimum data set.
4 The number of groups defined should be reasonably few (i.e. a few hundred rather than thousands) and they should cover all episodes without overlap (i.e. be exhaustive and mutually exclusive).

These criteria are useful as a guide, and some of them are easy to apply (exhaustiveness, exclusiveness, based on routine data). Others however are subjective (clinical similarity, relatively few) or are relative (statistical homogeneity).

In most cases, the subjective criteria have been applied through consensus panels, and this is as true of the original development of Diagnosis Related Groups (DRGs) as it has been of subsequent refinements of DRGs, both in the USA, Canada and Australia,[6] and in England. These consensus panels have used clinical opinion, but inevitably, opinions have varied as to whether a particular group is clinically homogeneous, and also as to the appropriate number of groups overall. These differences have led to much inconclusive debate, since there are no agreed objective standards which can be applied.

As a result, much of the emphasis in determining whether one grouping is better than another has depended on statistical criteria. The most usual statistic used has been based on the reduction in variance (RIV) of length of stay as a result of allocating episodes into groups.[7] In general, this has been a comparative process, seeking to obtain an improvement over a previous solution, rather than trying to achieve a particular standard of statistical homogeneity. Where available, hospital costs, or charges have also been used, but since most health care systems do not have detailed and accurate costing information, most of the work has been done using length of stay as a proxy for cost.

This emphasis has resulted in considerable amounts of sophisticated analysis, and considerable adjustment of the grouping criteria in order to gain small improvements in the statistical performance. Much work has also been done on adjusting the data sets as well, in order to overcome the problems posed by a few, very costly/long-stay episodes which have a significant effect on the estimate of the group means.

Development and use of diagnosis related groups in the USA

Diagnosis related groups were developed in the late 1960s at Yale University as a means of performance review and quality assurance. They have become the most widely known and implemented method of resource grouping, but are now largely used for costing and resource allocation and payment. In 1973, the first version was documented, which contained 333 groups, organized in 54 major diagnostic categories (MDCs). The second version, based on ICD 8, contained 83 MDCs and 383 DRGs, and the third version, developed for the State of New Jersey, was published in

1978. The final original version which contained 470 DRGs in 24 MDCs was completed in 1983 and was used as a basis of payment for all Medicare patients from October 1 1983.[8]

The allocation of patient episodes to a DRG starts by allocation to one of the 23 MDCs (which correspond to the body systems) on the basis of the primary diagnosis. Within an MDC, the episode is then allocated either to a surgical DRG, if there is a procedure, on the basis of that procedure, or, otherwise to a medical DRG on the basis of the primary diagnosis. In some instances, there is a further subdivision to a high- or low-cost group on the basis of the age of the patient (typically above or below 70 years) or the presence of certain complicating or co-morbid secondary diagnoses.

Since 1983, DRGs have evolved and been refined in a number of different ways. One stream of development has been through the DRGs used by the Health Care Financing Administration (HCFA) which has annually modified the DRGs used for Medicare payments in order to respond to changing patterns of care and diseases. A separate stream of development however has arisen from the perception that because of the Medicare programme, the HCFA DRGs have too much of a focus on elderly patients. This resulted in work in the late 1980s to develop a broader focus of the DRGs. The New York DRGs and CHAMPUS DRGs (Civilian Health and Medical Program of the Uniformed Services) were developed which sought a broader balance across all age groups, and the NACHRI grouper (National Association of Children's Hospitals and Related Institutions) which had a more specialized paediatric emphasis. These various initiatives came together in the production of the All Payer DRGs (APDRGs) in 1990, which have also been subsequently modified annually.

A separate strand of activity was also set up in the late 1980s in response to the criticisms that DRGs were not sufficiently sensitive to variations in severity of disease in patients. A number of ways of combining severity measures (such as using disease staging[9] or clinical severity[10]) were examined, and further work at Yale resulted in the Refined DRGs, in which levels of severity were assigned to each group of Adjacent DRGs (three levels in medical DRGs, and four levels in Surgical) resulting in about 1200 final groups. These levels of severity were identified by specific secondary diagnoses. The large number of groups in the refined DRGs model has meant that it has not been widely adopted, but the model continues to be available as an all payer refined (APR) DRG grouper.

There were a number of early competitors to the DRG model for classifying hospital activity mix, but the adoption of DRGs by HCFA has meant that all of these have had a minor role. One of the most interesting, in terms of exploring a different model, was the Patient Management Categories (PMCs) development, which was based on Patient Management

Pathways.[11] This started from the concept of types of patient conditions, and identified the typical resources associated with their care in the hospital sector, in order to identify the PMC. This is close to the concepts involved in the HBG/HRG matrix discussed in Chapter 1, but is confined to the care provided within the hospital, based on the context of care in the USA. Despite these shortcomings, the concepts of actual and potential multiple assignment, and making an explicit link between the condition and the activity are very helpful.

Development and use of resource groups outside the USA

During the '80s and '90s, the growing pressures on health care finances in all countries stimulated the search for ways to understand activity and costs. The DRG methodology was used as an example by many other countries and many of them explored the potential, and implemented DRGs or closely related variants, both for internal hospital management, and for financing hospital services.[12]

Various combinations of HCFA DRGs, APDRGs and AP refined DRGs have been implemented in different countries including Portugal, Ireland, Sweden and Spain, and detailed case studies of the implementation are available.[13] In most instances, the DRG methodology has been imported without modification, although the version of DRGs implemented varies between country, but in a number of instances, modifications to the DRG grouper have been undertaken to a greater or lesser extent.

In Canada, a rolling development programme of CMGs (casemix groups) has been undertaken by the Canadian Institute for Health Information (CIHI). This work started by using DRGs, and each MDC has been reviewed by clinical panels over a period of years and whilst keeping to the same basic design criteria, has resulted in substantially modified groupings. Similarly in Australia, the Australian National DRG (ANDRG) development programme has been based both on statistical and clinical review of the APDRG groupings, and has resulted in many minor and a number of substantial modifications.[14]

Minor modifications to DRGs have been undertaken in France to produce the Groupe Homogene de Malade (GHM)[15] and in Hungary, there have similarly been a small number of minor modifications in the development of a local variant, Homogen Betegseg Csoportok (HBKs).[16]

The exception to this process of adapting the DRG methodology to a local situation is in Germany where work has explored the use of PMCs as a way of categorizing patient activity.[17]

Development of resource groups in England

The trial application of DRGs in England occurred first in 1982/83,[18] but was more systematically applied in the Resource Management Programme in 1988/89.[19,20] This application involved collaboration with clinical directors, who accepted the general purpose of DRGs, but were unhappy with the clinical meaningfulness of the DRGs in English clinical practice. Although this criterion was subjective, it was felt to be important to address this issue by modifying the groupings in response to these clinical directors' advice. Consequently, in 1990, panels of clinical advisers (similar to those used by the Australian Clinical Casemix Committee) were set up to consider the construction of DRGs, and revise them where appropriate. Since then this has resulted in three versions of HRGs, released in 1992, 1994[21] and 1997[22] respectively.

The clinical working groups are made up of clinicians who have an interest in the issue, and the leader is nominated by the relevant specialty association in order to ensure that the resulting groups will be acceptable to the clinical professions as a whole. The recommendations are based upon their clinical expertise and statistical analysis of hospital inpatient data. The criteria used in the development were similar to those described for the development of DRGs:

- similar use of resources (as judged by length of stay)
- clinical meaningfulness
- relatively few (i.e. not more than 50 in one specialty area)
- based on items in the discharge minimum data set.

Data analysis was based on the discharge data set for England, about ten million episodes per year, including day cases. Tables of the mean and median lengths of stay by diagnosis and procedure were provided for each working group, together with various statistical analyses, including Reduction in Variance (RIV)* and Classification and Regression Tree Analysis (CART)[23] which was undertaken to provide an assessment of where the greatest improvements could be expected. In some instances it was clear that length of stay was not necessarily a good indicator of total cost so, where possible, other information on theatre, investigation, drug, disposables, etc. costs, was used to supplement the analysis. This has meant that

---

*The Reduction in Variance is a measure of the degree to which the variance in length of stay of the whole population can be explained by the variance between the means of the subgroups within the population. A high RIV means that most of the variance in cases is due to variance between the groups. A low RIV indicates that most of the population variance is within the groups.

Table 2.1: Reduction in variance due to DRGs and HRGs using English data, 1994/95

Grouper	RIV (%)
DRG Version 4 (1988)	28.6
HRG Version 1.1 (1992)	25.0
HRG Version 2 (1994)	32.2
HRG Version 3 (1997)	35.0

Table 2.2: Reduction in variance due to APDRGs and HRGs using Welsh data, 1995/96

LoS excluded (episodes)	APDRG (Wales Version 1997) (%)	HRG Version 2 (%)	HRG Version 3 (%)
>50 days	29.21	30.26	33.52
>100 days	27.11	27.18	30.06

sometimes length of stay information has been over-ridden, based upon clinical views and other costing information.

No single gold standard exists with which to compare the performance of HRGs, but comparison with a standard DRG grouper and the refined DRG grouper provides some indication of the amount of homogeneity that can be expected. Table 2.1 shows a comparison of HRGs; Version 1, Version 2 and Version 3 with DRGs 1988, and Table 2.2 shows a comparison of HRGs with the APDRG grouper used in Wales (APDRG Version 1997). In the last seven years, a steady improvement in the explanation of variance in length of stay has been achieved through enabling the clinical working groups to focus on areas in which there is the greatest potential for improvement. This shows that Version 3 HRGs can provide an improved reduction of variance of length of stay for English hospital data and that for Welsh hospital data, Version 2 was slightly better, but Version 3 HRGs substantially better than APDRGs. Of course this may not be true for other countries for which the grouping algorithms have not been optimized.

The proposed HRGs are agreed through a process of consultation with the NHS and through specialty assurance provided by the relevant colleges and specialty associations. The proposals are also discussed with the Joint Consultants Committee which is the formal interface between the hospital specialists and the Department of Health. Final specifications of the groupings are then drawn up and released to the NHS together with software for allocating records into HRGs and appropriate documentation.

The structure of HRGs Version 3

In Version 3 HRGs there are 572 groups organized in 19 chapters (one of which is for invalid records) and these are mainly body system/clinical specialty orientated. The groupings are allocated on the basis of procedure, primary diagnosis, secondary diagnosis, age and discharge status and the diagnostic codes use ICD 9 or ICD 10 (for data collected after April 1995). The groupings are exhaustive and exclusive, in other words, there is only one appropriate group for any particular record and every record can be allocated to a group. Seven 'U' groups are used to cover various errors in data quality in diagnoses, procedures or age values.

A case is allocated to a final HRG through a number of steps.

- The first check is to determine whether a valid diagnosis is present. If not the case is allocated to a 'U' group.
- If a procedure code is present, the record will be grouped directly into the appropriate surgical group.
- Records with more than one procedure code are checked using a procedure hierarchy to see which is the most costly procedure. The record is allocated to an HRG on that basis. The final procedure grouping may also be influenced by the presence of a secondary diagnosis or by the age of the patient.
- Records without procedures are allocated to medical groups on the basis of primary diagnosis, although this may also be modified by the presence of a secondary diagnosis or age.

The procedure hierarchy is used to ensure that the most resource intensive procedure is used for grouping irrespective of its position within the record. All OPCS4 codes have been allocated a rank based upon the average length of stay in the primary position. A value of zero is allocated to procedures which are deemed to be non-operative and these are ignored for the purpose of grouping, and the record is therefore grouped by diagnosis.

Secondary diagnoses may also be used to indicate complications or comorbidity and elevate a case into a higher cost group. Lists of complications and comorbidities are, in general, chapter specific and in some instances, are specific to a single HRG. Similarly, the age splits used are usually above/below 70 years, but in some instances 65, 75 or other ages are used.

Version 3 HRGs have introduced new chapters for spinal procedures and vascular surgery (chapters R and Q respectively), and the redefinition of a number of minor investigative procedures (especially endoscopies) allows a better separation of short-stay episodes for investigation from those longer episodes in which investigation and treatment are combined.

Other changes have been the introduction of complex medical elderly HRGs within each chapter, and a separate group for holiday relief.

Healthcare Resource Groups have been criticized by some observers for departing from the original method of construction. In particular, it has been suggested that developing an alternative set of groups prevents the possibility of international comparisons. In practice this is not an issue, in part because different countries have implemented different and non-comparable versions of DRGs, and also because records can always be grouped to a standard DRG version, provided that they have been collected with ICD diagnoses and procedure codes which can be mapped to ICD 9–clinical modification. In any case, cross-national comparisons, although interesting to the academic community, because of the variations in clinical traditions and organization of care, have rarely produced useful results for policy or performance management. It is of course true that developing a local grouper is expensive, but this is offset by the potential gain due to improved efficiency. Moreover, this investment is helpful in encouraging the local ownership of clinicians and managers who are the people who will have to use the casemix groups.

Further development of inpatient resource groups

The statistical techniques used in the last ten years to help refine both DRGs and HRGs have resulted in groupings which will be difficult to improve given the quality of data and limitations of data sets. Part of this is due to the inherent variation in any large data set due to differences in clinical practice, and the availability of resources in different places. There is however another problem in groupings of treatment episodes (both for DRGs and HRGs) which is that non-surgical episodes are based on the diagnosis, rather than the activity undertaken. Because clinical care varies, the treatment and cost for a particular condition may differ from place to place. The move towards activity-based groupings to deal with this issue is discussed below.

Outpatient and community groupings

Unlike inpatient episodes, data sets for capturing activity outside hospital are not widely available, and methods of grouping have been much less intensively developed. However, if we are to manage the whole of the health service properly, it is crucial to be able to monitor and measure activity in all sectors. The experience in the USA of the explosion of ambulatory costs following the introduction of prospective payment for inpatients based on DRGs is a warning that trying to manage one sector without being able to manage others is likely to have unforeseen effects. As a consequence of this, a number of efforts to capture and classify ambulatory activity have been undertaken in the USA. These include ambulatory visit groups (AVGs),[24] in which the design criteria were similar to DRGs in that the primary diagnosis was used to allocate the episode to a chapter. In a subsequent development, ambulatory procedure groups (APGs),[25] the use of diagnosis was dropped, and the grouping was driven entirely by procedure. These approaches are even more culture specific than inpatient groupings, and there has been little enthusiasm for adopting them in other countries. Part of the difficulty is that the consultation aspect of outpatient attendances in the UK does not result in a surgical procedure in most instances, nor is the model appropriate to the grouping of community services where care is either aimed at prevention (particularly health visiting) or at the long-term support and care of individuals with irreversible disease and disability. In this latter instance, care is being provided by nurses or by professionals such as physiotherapists, occupational therapists, etc.

Just as difficult is the lack of data sets collected in outpatient or community service settings. Although an outpatient data set is now collected in England, this does not yet contain procedure or diagnosis information. Discussions on a community minimum data set have been undertaken in England over a number of years, however a satisfactory data set has yet to be agreed or implemented. In addition, proposals for the management of community services through Primary Care Groups/Trusts are likely to delay the implementation of an agreed data set. (Mental health also presents problems which are discussed in Chapter 4.)

Not only is there a shortage of useful models for grouping out-of-hospital care, there are constraints to the development of better groupings of interventions which are common to all sectors and these are discussed below.

Activity definitions

To be consistent, a set of resource groups should be defined on the basis of a package of activity being undertaken. For simplicity's sake this also means that there should be one main activity that is the cost driver, and which reasonably accurately predicts the costs of all the other components of care. This condition is met mainly in surgical episodes, where the surgical procedure is not only the most costly item, but also predicts the amount of pre- and post-operative care required. This may also be true for some procedure-based outpatient contacts, and also in community settings where particular nursing procedures are undertaken.

For other episodes of care (both within and outside of hospital) however the description of the activity undertaken may not be so straightforward or one-dimensional. Furthermore, surgical procedures are classified and collected as routine hospital statistics, but other activities (whether medical, nursing or investigational) are not.

Not only is non-surgical activity not widely captured, there are no classifications of non-surgical activity available. This has meant that in order to develop activity groupings which describe the resources used, where there is no procedure, DRGs (and HRGs) have been based upon the diagnosis on the assumption that patients with particular diagnoses receive similar packages of care. Thus, the prediction of cost is based not on the activity delivered, but on the activity *expected* to be delivered for this type of patient. If this varies considerably between different places or clinicians, then the accuracy of the prediction of cost will be poor. This has been a particular feature of the problems involved in groupings for mental health episodes of care,[26] as diagnosis in particular is a very poor predictor of the care package provided. Even when modified by other descriptions of the patient's condition (social functioning, etc.) there is great variability in the package and cost of care provided.

As a corollary, these kinds of resource group, since they are based on the condition as a proxy for activity undertaken, cannot be used in conjunction with condition groups to determine the appropriateness of care. For example, in a surgical specialty, it is possible to identify that for patients with appendicitis, appendicectomy is an appropriate treatment, however, for medical patients with a myocardial infarction, the resource group 'myocardial infarction' is not useful in determining whether an appropriate package of care was provided. Inevitably, quite a large proportion of health care (i.e. all non-surgical activity) is currently subject to this difficulty. Mental health and elderly care are large specialty areas which are bound to suffer from this difficulty and for which proxies have had to be used in the absence of detailed and consistent activity data.

Because of this problem, much of the acute inpatient casemix literature is confused about the difference between groupings of conditions and groupings of activities, so much so, that the most widely known grouping, DRGs, although being based on treatment episodes, suggests in its name, that it is a grouping of patients with similar diagnoses.

Other grouping systems have less ambiguity, Disease Staging for instance is clearly about stages of condition, Ambulatory Procedure Groups are clearly groupings of procedures and the HRGs signal the purpose of the groups in relation to resources.

Paradoxically, although the development of coding and minimum data sets in community services is much less well-developed than for inpatients, it has been easier to incorporate descriptions of activity into proposed data sets. Indeed, the concept of care packages, care profiles and pathways is much better understood in community services, and this work provides a natural pathway towards developing activity-based groupings for community services. Even this however will not solve the problem of multiple-cost drivers and across all health care activities it will be necessary to combine diagnostic activity, nursing and medical/pharmacological interventions, rather than just being able to use surgical procedure as the main resource driver.

Definitions of episodes

Activity-based resource groups depend upon the concept that there are consistent patterns of activity within a treatment episode. If it is impossible to define the episode consistently, then the concept of a consistent pattern of activity is clearly difficult. Episodes of hospital care can be fairly readily standardized, since the start and end point are clear. Problems arise when patients are transferred to a different unit for specific components of care (such as intensive care or convalescence), or when the care is provided in a number of discrete admissions, such as chemotherapy, or haemodialysis. Much more difficult however are the definitions of care outside hospital, both in hospital-based ambulatory settings (e.g. outpatient visits, ward attendances, domiciliary visits, etc.) and in community care. In these situations, there are real difficulties in identifying when an episode starts and finishes, and there may be several different types of contact and episode running concurrently. In the mental health specialty, care may be provided intermittently, and lapse for several months before being resumed, if ever.

Current work aimed at producing a consistent definition of episode across sectors proposes four levels of episode to describe health care activity:

- *Problem episode* which describes all the health care interventions administered for a specific problem and may include care from several providers and/or care teams.
- *Provider episode* which describes all the health care interventions for a particular problem, administered by one provider only (but may involve one or more care teams).
- *Care episode* which describes all the health care interventions administered by one care team for a specific problem.

- *Care element* which describes one element (contact, visit, attendance, bed-day, etc.) of health care intervention provided by one health care professional.

This approach is intended to enable the final development of episode definition across all sectors to maintain a consistent conceptual base, although obviously there are differences between community and acute care in the key factors which naturally define start and end points. For example, for some conditions such as Learning Disability the only logical start and end points of care may be time related, whereas for some acute conditions such as appendicitis, start and end points based on admission and discharge can be clearly defined.

The above approach however does allow for those conditions which require combinations of acute and community care. Not only does this require new definitions of contacts and episode types, but it also requires the ability to link contacts across time, and potentially across providers. This will of course be greatly assisted by the development of a unique patient identifier, such as the NHS number.

Because these problems are difficult does not mean that they are impossible to solve, nor does it mean that they have to be ignored; however the challenge of producing useful groupings, not only of activities, but of the contacts within an episode remains one to be addressed. In a sense, this is a grouping problem, not of defining similar types of episodes of care, but of grouping contacts/episodes within the career of a patient, so that the overall episodes of care are similar.[27]

Minimum data sets

A further problem in the development of activity data is that although minimum data sets for hospitalization of patients have been routinely collected in most countries for many years, this is not true of outpatient or community-based care. It is much more difficult to collect data on these patients because they are cared for in dispersed places, and the clerical back-up which exists in hospitals is often absent. This means that health care professionals have to collect data for what appears to be a bureaucratic exercise, without proper support or training, and with very little useful feedback of the data. In some health systems of course these data are collected as a part of the reimbursement process and, without careful safeguards, the potential for distortion and corruption of these data is substantial.

Not only are there organizational difficulties in collecting data, but the data are difficult to collect as well. Many patients receiving community care have multiple conditions so the definition of a primary diagnosis is difficult, and in any case, the pathological diagnosis may be less important than the patient's condition, level of support by carers, and ability to look after themselves. All of this means that in some sectors the use of a diagnostic label is not perceived as useful, however, achieving agreement by different professional groups on the classification of functions and disabilities may be difficult. In addition, the definitions of activities undertaken are problematic, particularly in relation to deciding what is important enough to collect, and what is not.

Many countries are developing ways of capturing this type of information,[28] but the ideal would be to develop patient-based information systems in which electronic records replace the paper forms, and then enable the capture of the statistical information as a by-product of direct patient care. Few countries have yet developed systematic patient-based information in community-based services. This means that not only are there gaps in the knowledge of the care of particular types of patients outside hospitals, but it is difficult to identify bundles of care that span the inpatient and outpatient settings and develop and monitor integrated services.

For example, patients with strokes are often admitted to an acute medical ward, and after a few days, which include diagnostic tests and stabilization, transferred to a rehabilitation programme. This programme may be delivered in the same ward, in a rehabilitation unit in the same hospital, in a different hospital, or in a community-based 'hospital-at-home' service. All of these make up a very similar package of care, but unless the community care element is recorded, those units which deliver the care via the community look extremely efficient compared to other units. This is because their length of stay is short, suggesting low resource use in hospital, but the compensating resources that they used in the community are not identified.

Until the community/outpatient element of care can be captured and grouped satisfactorily, comparisons of the relative efficiency of different hospitals are always likely to be potentially misleading.

Applications of casemix groupings in health service management

As discussed in Chapter 1, the use of groupings of patients and treatment episodes could support the assessment of needs of the population and the consequent resource requirements, together with monitoring the appropriateness of care and the outcomes achieved. However, the development of condition groups which are robust and usable across the whole health care spectrum has some way to go before all the potential can be realized. For this reason, the applications discussed in Chapters 5 to 9 in this book will focus on the use of HRGs. These cover application from a GP and health authority perspective, as well as use within a provider at trust and individual clinical directorate level. In addition, the potential of using HRGs, not just for examining costs, but also to provide some insight into potential quality issues is discussed in Chapter 7.

References

1   DHSS (1968) *Report on Hospital Inpatient Enquiry, Historical Tables for the years 1949, 1957–62.* HMSO, London.
2   Benjamin B (1965) Hospital Activity Analyses. An information feedback for the consultant. *The Hospital* 61: 221–8.
3   Roger France FH (1993) Hospital Information Systems in Europe: Trends towards uniformity in patient record summaries. In *Diagnosis Related Groups in Europe, Uses and Perspectives* (eds M Casas and MM Wiley). Springer-Verlag, Berlin.
4   Office of Population Census and Surveys (1990) *Classification of Surgical Operations and Procedures.* 4th revision. HMSO, London.
5   Fetter RB, Shin Y, Freeman JL *et al.* (1980) Casemix definition by Diagnosis Related Group. *Medical Care* 18 (**Suppl. 1–53**): 1–53.
6   Pilla J and Hindle D (1994) Adapting DRGs, the British, Canadian and Australian experiences. *Australian Health Information Management* 24: 87–93.
7   McGuire TE (1991) DRGs: The state of the art circa 1990. *Health Policies* 17: 97–119.
8   McGuire TE (1993) DRG evolution. In *Diagnosis Related Groups in Europe, Uses and Perspectives* (eds M Casas and MM Wiley). Springer-Verlag, Berlin.
9   Gonella JS, Hornbrook MC and Louis DZ (1984) Staging of Disease: a casemix measurement. *JAMA* 241: 637–44.
10 Horn SD and Sharkey PD (1983) Severity of Illness to Predict Patient Resource Use within DRGs. *Inquiry* 20: 314–21.
11 Young WW, Swinkola RB and Zorn DM (1982) The Measurement of Hospital Casemix. *Medical Care* 20: 501–12.
12 Kimberly JR and de Pourville G (eds) (1993) *The Migration of Managerial Innovation. Diagnosis related groups and health care administration in Western Europe.* Jossey Bass, San Francisco.
13 Casas M and Wiley MM (eds) (1993) *Diagnosis Related Groups in Europe, Uses and Perspectives.* Springer-Verlag, Berlin.

14 Pilla J and Hindle D (1994) *Op cit.*

15 de Pourville G (1993) France: the introduction of casebased hospital management. In *The Migration of Managerial Innovation. Diagnosis related groups and health care administration in Western Europe* (eds JR Kimberly and G de Pourville). Jossey Bass, San Francisco.

16 Bordas I, Nagy J and Karolyi Z (1995) *Refining the Hungarian Healthcare System using a Classification System.* Proceedings of 11th International PCSE Conference. pp. 184–94.

17 Neubauer G (1993) Germany: an outsider in DRG development. In *The Migration of Managerial Innovation. Diagnosis related groups and health care administration in Western Europe* (eds JR Kimberly and G de Pourville). Jossey Bass, San Francisco.

18 Sanderson HF and Andrews V (1984) Monitoring hospital services: an application of DRGs to hospital discharge data in England and Wales. *Occasional Paper, London School of Hygiene and Tropical Medicine*, June. London.

19 Sanderson H, Craig M, Winyard G *et al.* (1986) Using Diagnosis Related Groups in the NHS. *Community Medicine* **8, No. 1**: 37–47.

20 Sanderson HF, Storey A, Morris D *et al.* (1989) Evaluation of Diagnosis Related Groups in the National Health Service. *Community Medicine* **11, No. 4**: 269–78.

21 Sanderson HF, Anthony P and Mountney LM (1995) Health care Resource Groups Version 2. *Journal of Public Health Medicine* **17(3)**: 349–54.

22 NHS Executive (1997) *HRGs Version 3.* National Casemix Office, Winchester.

23 Breiman L, Friedman JH, Olshen RA *et al.* (1984) *Classification and Regression Trees.* Wadsworth International Group. Chapman & Hall, London.

24 Schneider KC, Lichtenstein JL, Fetter RB *et al.* (1991) *The new ICD-9-CM Ambulatory Visit Groups Classification Scheme. Definitions Manual 1986.* Yale University, New Haven, CT.

25 Hutchinson A, Parkin D and Philips P (1991) Casemix Measures for Ambulatory Care. *Journal of Public Health Medicine* **13**: 189–97.

26 Taube CA, Lee ES, Forthofer RN (1984) DRGs in psychiatry: an empirical evaluation. *Medical Care* **22(7)**: 597–610.

27 Rigby M, Severs M, Swayne J *et al.* (1994) Time to Outlaw the episode? *British Journal of Healthcare Computing* **11**: 26–8.

28 Eager K (1997) *SNAP project report.* University of Wollongong, New South Wales.

3   Condition groupings

Introduction

As described in Chapter 2, the four-level model of health care is an important device to help make sense of the response of the health care systems to individuals in need. As we have described in Chapter 2 on resource groupings, by far the most development work has been undertaken at the diagnosed disease/ curative services level, because this fits well with the ICD, and the higher-cost services. Whilst this emphasis is understandable in terms of dealing with the most expensive areas, it does not address the fundamental issues of comprehensive planning of health care, and the balance between the role of high-volume/low-cost primary care services and the high-cost/low-volume secondary care sector. In order to get a comprehensive view of patient care, it is important to ensure that a wider view of conditions is explored, including at-risk states, symptomatic presentations and functional limitations.

Design criteria and issues

Like resource groups, condition groups need to have criteria for their design in order to judge whether the proposed groupings are satisfactory. However, the key criterion of similarity of condition is much more difficult to define and measure.

Two main potential uses exist for similar condition groups, either to predict the intervention required, or to predict the outcome. Of these two characteristics, the latter is easier to measure if there is an easily measured outcome, such as death or a well-validated physiological measure, symptom or function scale, and in some conditions (such as cancers) good information about the prognosis is available which has been used to classify stages and grades of tumours. This is not however true across the whole range of conditions. Many conditions are less severe, and the outcome is not death, but discomfort/disability. In these instances, measurement of outcome is more subjective and less certain.

Casemix groupings for the purpose of predicting the risk of an adverse outcome may be based on diagnosis, but there will be many instances where other characteristics of the patient are very important. Variables such as age, availability of family support, performance status, and especially for critically ill patients, scores based on physiological measures, such as Apache, Medisgrps, Severity Groups, can be collapsed into a small number of severity grades which can be used to predict mortality or adverse outcome. In some instances, such as Apache, these can be completely independent of the pathological diagnosis. Whereas, in the staging of a cancer, the variables predicting outcome are additional to the diagnosis.

Prediction of intervention however is much more dependent upon the diagnosis or problem statement and subjective. It is based on what a particular clinician will judge that it is right to do under certain clinical conditions and it may differ from clinician to clinician, depending upon training, availability of resources, and also on the general condition of the patient. There is of course information on the appropriate care for particular conditions from textbooks and journals, and increasingly from clinical guidelines and evidence-based medicine. There is however still debate over many conditions, and evidence-based advice to cover the whole spectrum of illness to develop comprehensive condition groupings is not yet available.

Development of condition groupings at present therefore is based on two approaches, the statistical testing of patient data to identify predictors of outcome (which may be independent of diagnosis) and the development of diagnosis/condition-based groupings which predict clinical interventions, but based on clinical opinions and expertise, and where available, evidence-based practice.

Existing developments

Both aspects of condition groups have been important in the developments in the USA and elsewhere. Iso-prognosis groupings have been developed which can be used to adjust for the expected outcome of disease, and for quality assurance/audit, and iso-severity groupings which can predict the likely requirement for care, and hence explain increased cost of care. It is the latter aspect that has driven most of the development in the USA, as researchers have sought to find a suitable severity adjuster to add on to DRGs, as a way of predicting and allocating costs,[1,2] but in addition, ways of defining the care required, or to be made available, for the population, have also been explored.[3]

This section reviews briefly a number of approaches to the issue of condition classification, and starts with general schemes, which aim to cover the whole spectrum of disease (at least that within the ICD), but also covers some specialized classifications for particular types of patient.

Disease staging

One of the best known, and most durable condition grouping methods is disease staging, which grew out of the concepts of staging of disease in cancer.[4] (This is itself of course a type of condition grouping, widely used in comparisons of outcomes of cancer treatments.) In disease staging, approximately 420 diagnostic categories are divided into four main stages (and a variable number of sub-stages), depending upon the severity and degree of progression of the condition. The scheme is based on ICD, and coded staging uses primary and secondary diagnosis codes. Clinical staging also uses physiological and other clinical data to define more precise stages and sub-stages. Disease staging has been used for predicting resource use (as a modifier for DRGs), and also as a severity adjuster for comparisons of mortality rates.[5] A further application has used disease stage as a marker of the appropriateness of location of care,[6] and, like the primary-care sensitive conditions, can be used to identify cases which should have been cared for in primary care and not in hospital. Development and updating of disease staging has been carried out over a number of years.

Patient management categories

Patient management categories are groupings of conditions based upon patient management pathways (PMPs).[7] They were developed by panels of clinicians and within each major condition area, identify a number of types of presentation, assessment processes, and treatment pathways. Each major condition area (chapter) is thus broken up into a number of pathways, and management groups. These groups are clinically and statistically homogeneous, and combine a grouping of the condition with the treatment. They have been used for a number of purposes, including prediction of resource use (cost) as an alternative to DRGs, and as tools for quality assurance and audit, comparing actual treatment pathways with those expected, and actual outcomes with those expected.

Development of PMCs has been halted, but the assignment software continues to be available for research purposes. Although this has not been widely used outside the USA, there has been work to develop the PMC approach for managing health services in Germany.[8]

Coded/clinical severity

An alternative approach to the development of condition groups grew out of the work on global measures of health status undertaken in the 1970s in which indicators of risk of death, or poor outcome were identified, and used to construct pathology-independent indices of severity of illness.[9] These mainly required detailed clinical information, not available in the hospital discharge abstract, and this was the origin of the work undertaken to develop clinical severity. Because of the cost of capturing this information, it has only had a limited impact outside of the USA, but in some studies, the extra information has proved useful in comparing the outcomes of care, and variations in costs of care.[10]

Medisgrps

A similar approach pioneered in Massachusetts resulted in the development of Medisgrps,[11] in which a similar set of variables used in a proprietary algorithm enabled patients to be allocated to differing severity groupings. Like clinical severity, the increased amount of information required, which needed to be captured by trained abstracters, has proved to be prohibitively expensive for use outside of the USA, and an evaluation in England showed the technique to be of little value in the NHS.[12]

Oregon condition/treatment pairs

A different need led to the development of condition/treatment pairs in the Oregon Experiment.[13] The intention was to find a way of rationing care provided by the Medicaid programme. The condition/treatment pairs were ranked in level of importance and priority by members of the community. The condition groups were constructed around the ICD, and the treatments based on hospital care. In this sense, it was a limited description of the complete process of care (excluding preventive, investigative, caring and supportive functions), although it probably focused on the major cost components of care. Although the basis of the groupings was logical, the application in the USA for developing rationing decisions has resulted in little development of the condition-grouping process. However, a development of this process, with resource modelling has been undertaken in the Illawarrogon project in New South Wales.

Burden-of-disease groupings

In a similar way, but for the purpose of assisting in the allocation of resources in developing country settings, work has been undertaken by WHO to identify the global burdens of disease.[14] Again, the condition groupings are based on ICD, and the interventions, preventive and curative, are identified as health programmes. This systematic approach allows an appraisal of the most cost-effective way to deploy scarce health service resources.

Patient-related groups

The requirement of funding area population-based services in Hong Kong has led to development of condition/treatment-based grouping systems, on which the resources required for care can be based. These groups are linked to evidence-based protocols, with specified outcome indicators, and are intended to cover the complete episode of care across hospital, outpatient and community care. This approach is being developed on a rolling basis with the intention of eventually covering those conditions which are most important in resource terms.[15]

Ambulatory care groups

Work by a group from Johns Hopkins Medical School[16] aimed at classifying the types of conditions and interventions seen in primary care, has resulted in the development of a two-stage grouping. The first step is based on diagnosis and results in a classification of 34 ambulatory diagnostic groups. The activities associated with these are then further classified (including multiple visits) into a set of 51 ambulatory care groups which are intended to be similar in resource use.

Specialized classifications

The purpose of this chapter is to review ways of classifying the whole spectrum of health conditions, but some of the particular approaches for specific groups could be considered. In some instances, it might be appropriate to incorporate these methods into a broader system, or at least to learn lessons from the methods that have been used. However, it is not possible to review here all of the specific severity scoring systems which have been developed.

Comprehensive condition groups

In all of these developments of groupings of types of patients, the main emphasis has been on classifying patients who present to the health care system in order to assess their care requirements, or their likely prognosis. Most of the systems are based on diagnosis, those which are not, use physiological measures, or in some instances assessments of functional ability.

For the purpose of identifying the comprehensive care requirements of a population there are difficulties in integrating these groupings across the whole spectrum of conditions (i.e. not just diagnoses), and in general they also lack a population perspective. This is a problem if there is significant unmet need that is not presented for health care (especially in the social and economically disadvantaged sections of the community) or need which is inappropriately presented and met.

The extensive literature on variations in utilization rates, and medical practice, illustrates the need for a way of understanding how the morbidity in the population is met by health services if there is to be equity (geographical and social) in the availability of care.[17] One way to help this understanding is to classify all of the conditions in the population, so that they can be compared with the appropriate interventions and provide an assessment of the degree of fit between the care provided and the care expected.

A systematic way of undertaking this has been sought for some time, programme planning approaches by WHO over many years have resulted in a number of piecemeal developments.[18] Similarly, programme budgeting developments have been pursuing a similar course.[19] These seek to develop truly comprehensive views of the health of the population and the options for providing care, and thus need to be able to classify the complete spectrum of care. The difficulty of course is the lack of comprehensive and reliable information. What there is, is usually based on ICD, so most classifications have been based mainly on this, but there is a risk of underestimating the services required for the prevention of disease in individuals at-risk, the needs for diagnostic assessment in those who have symptoms, but in whom the diagnosis is eventually excluded, and those with chronic and irreversible disease, for whom the issue is not seeking a cure, but the requirements for care and support to ameliorate disability, discomfort and distress.

To deal with this comprehensive approach to planning and providing care requires the four-level model of care described in Chapter 1, and although this may not be appropriate for all health care systems, the systematic use of information to understand the morbidity of the population and the services required has substantial potential for delivering appropriate and equitable services.

Health Benefit Groups

The purpose of the development of condition groups in England was to develop groupings which helped purchasers and providers to understand the complete spectrum of care for a particular problem, and in which the implications of disease could be described in terms of HRGs. In this development it has been necessary to look wider than the ICD, in order to deal with potential disease, as well as disabling and chronic conditions. This means that the classification will require data that are not yet systematically available, but which could in time be available from electronic clinical records. This also means that the HBGs are a distinctly different phase of development from previous classifications of conditions in that, although comprehensive, they are not immediately applicable, but they will be able to use information from clinical systems, both in primary and secondary care, when these have been sufficiently widely implemented.

Unlike other classifications of conditions, HBGs are constructed around the four separate, but related, areas of classification, as follows.

At-risk

These HBGs relate to condition states of individuals who are presently healthy, but who have a predisposition to develop a condition. This may be due to a genetic factor (e.g. familial polyposis coli, predisposing to cancer of the colon), or an environmental or behavioural factor (e.g. asbestos exposure, tobacco smoker). These risk factors may predispose to one specific disease or a number of diseases (for instance tobacco smoking may lead to lung cancer, chronic bronchitis and emphysema, coronary heart disease, peripheral vascular disease, etc.) The interventions associated with these at-risk states may be classed as health promotion, often to groups, or to the population as a whole, seeking to promote healthy behaviour or prevention, in which the activity is focused on individuals, aiming to prevent specific conditions (such as immunization for those without immunity to certain bacterial or viral diseases). In some instances, this includes screening, where the detection of early, or premalignant changes may be able to prevent subsequent development of invasive cancer. In other instances, screening enables early diagnosis but is not strictly prevention aimed at changing an at-risk state. Clearly, there are some conditions for which there is no appropriate preventive care available. In those instances, there is no need to specify at-risk conditions, since there is no intervention required.

Symptomatic presentation

This is not an important area of HBGs for some conditions, where the investigation and assessment of patients is simple and cheap, and may be a part of the initiation of treatment. However, some conditions do require expensive investigation in order to confirm or exclude the diagnosis (especially where the diagnosis is life-threatening and the treatment expensive or risky), and planning and commissioning services need to provide for the appropriate level of diagnostic service. It is important to emphasize that many of those presenting with symptoms will be found not to have the particular condition, thus, the number of diagnostic services required will frequently be greater than the numbers of cases diagnosed. However, the reassurance of excluding a diagnosis is an important part of health services and needs to be funded and provided.

By their nature, these conditions cannot be classified by diagnosis (although there may be suitable symptom codes within the ICD), and symptoms and problem statements are more appropriate. Clearly, some symptoms may be associated with more than one diagnosis (e.g. chest pain, acute abdominal pain) and as in the at-risk area, one symptom-HBG may lead to more than one diagnosis-HBG. This is particularly true for the more generalized symptoms (malaise, weight loss, etc.) but is also true for more specific presentations, such as rectal bleeding, or a breast lump.

Diagnosed (reversible) disease

Most acute health care service is focused around this level of the HBGs, although much of the work of primary medical care may also deal with these conditions. The distinction between this level and the next (extensive/irreversible disease) is the objective of care, which at this level is concerned with cure or stabilization and returning the individual to as near normal health as possible. The appropriate classification is therefore the pathologically based diagnosis as in the ICD, which because reversal of the pathology is being attempted, is the key determinant of the services provided. For some diagnoses, the ICD does not have sufficient detail to predict the intervention (or the outcome) and more detail at a clinical level may be required. For example, in cancers, the stage is a crucial variable in defining the treatment applied, and also in predicting the likely outcome of care. Consequently, the information from existing routine information systems which are based on the ICD may not be sufficient, even if supplemented by the clinical modifications of ICD 9 CM.

Irreversible (chronic) disease

In contrast to the third level of groupings, where intervention is aimed at cure or stabilization, in the chronic and irreversible stage of disease, health services are aiming to provide care, support, relief from pain and discomfort, and as much normal functioning as is possible within the limits of the condition. The focus of the classification is therefore based, not on the pathology, but on the disability or discomfort, and the service required to minimize that. For example, patients with advanced cancer and with severe rheumatoid arthritis require pain relief, those with a stroke and those with head injuries require rehabilitation and aids to mobility.

Any individual however may have a condition that has pathology and functional dimensions, and if both aspects require care, then it will be important to make provision for the requirement, both of pathology-specific, as well as general supportive care. It is of course important to ensure that this does not result in double counting, especially from services that deliver general care and pathology-specific treatment.

Managing the information for HBGs

As noted earlier, there is little systematic information with which we can describe the epidemiology of the population. In principle, it would be desirable to have access to complete and detailed information on all the individuals in the population. From a purchasing/commissioning point of view, the requirement is to identify the numbers of individuals requiring care in the next year (or relevant time period) and the cost and expected outcome from that care. From a providers' perspective, it would be useful to be able to consider alternative ways of delivering the care for the individuals expected over the next year. From both these perspectives, the numbers should be based either on the yearly incidence (for symptoms and acute conditions), or on the period prevalence (for at-risk or chronic, long-term conditions). It is important to note that unlike HRGs, HBGs do not need to be mutually exclusive. It is possible for one individual to have more than one condition, and for those conditions to be receiving different packages of care. Hence, that individual may be in more than one HBG, but each package of care can only be in one HRG.

Developing epidemiological surveys of the population in order to assess the numbers of individuals in each HBG would be a very expensive and time-consuming exercise. Pilot studies have demonstrated that it is difficult with present sources of information to collect the detail to an adequate level (see Chapter 10). However, the information held by each GP on the individuals in their practice provides an alternative source of information. Although this is based on contact and may therefore still underestimate the true morbidity, it is much more likely to be complete than hospital activity data. General practitioner data have been collected in England for many years on a paper basis as the source material for the GP Morbidity Survey,[20] and this exercise is being taken forward as the Collection of Health Data from General Practice project. Pilots of the use of representative GPs with computer systems suggest that if properly managed and if all the participants agree a minimum data set, valuable epidemiological data can be collected at very low cost.[21]

Development and application

Because of the constraints of data, the development of HBGs is less advanced that that of HRGs, at least in acute inpatient care. However, HBGs for five initial areas (lung, colorectal and breast cancer, head injury, stroke, coronary heart disease and female sexual health), have been completed by multi-disciplinary working groups. These groups have consisted of GPs, public health physicians, hospital consultants, nurses (both hospital and community based) and allied health professionals. They have sought to identify the types of patients within each level of the HBG model, and have also described the potential interventions. The data have then been summarized as a matrix of the conditions and interventions. The definition of each of these groups has then been set out in Read-coded clinical terms, so that clinical information systems could, in theory, provide analyses of patient records in terms of HBGs.

These initial groupings have been tested in pilot sites, where partnerships of health authority, GP purchaser, and provider (acute and/or community) have sought to identify the numbers of individuals in each HBG and the numbers of episodes of care provided. This has led to discussions of how the service should be organized, and what the changes would imply in the costs and outcomes of care.

The conclusions of this exercise have reinforced the fact that at present it is very difficult to capture all the data required (epidemiological, activity and cost) but that the exercise of setting the process out systematically can be a useful way of organizing the process, and identifying what key information is missing. It was also clear that to undertake the exercise across the whole spectrum of conditions and care was beyond the capability of data collection or comprehension at this stage, although it was also recognized that moving towards a complete picture would be helpful over a longer period.

Integration

This description of the types of patients and the types of interventions, using a comprehensive model of health care, can provide not just a definition of the care required but also a way of monitoring the quality and effectiveness of care. The four levels of the HBG/HRG model can be used to identify the objectives of care, and the quality criteria (process and outcome) can be used to assess whether those objectives have been met.

As an example, the Appendix in Chapter 1 showed a summary matrix for breast cancer, with quality process and outcome indicators. The potential outcome indicators (technical and consumer) are listed in the right-hand column, and these apply to the four separate levels of the HBGs. The process indicators, appropriateness, equity, and efficiency are shown in the bottom rows, and relate to the relevant areas of HRGs. The implications of this integrated model are that it should be possible eventually to build clinical information systems to capture the complete clinical record (and which link seamlessly to other clinical records for the same patient) and from which key information can be derived to construct condition groups, intervention groups (for planning and commissioning) and structure, process and outcome indicators for monitoring to describe the performance of the system.

Although there are currently difficulties in collecting some of these quality measures, over time, as the quality of data improves, so will the quality of the outcome indicators. Similarly, if the model can be used to provide a structure for systematizing evidence-based medical interventions, then the appropriateness of care can be relatively easily monitored with the output of information from clinical systems.

References

1 Thomas JW and Ashcraft MLF (1991) Measuring Severity of Illness: Six severity systems and their ability to explain cost variations. *Inquiry* **28**: 39–55.

2 Horn SD and Sharkey PD (1983) Measuring Severity of Illness to Predict Patient Resource Use with DRGs. *Inquiry* **20**: 314–21.

3 Murray CJL and Lopez AD (eds) (1994) *Global Comparative Assessments in the Health Sector*. WHO, Geneva.

4 Gonnella JS, Hornbrook MC and Louis DZ (1984) Staging of Disease: A casemix measure. *Journal of the American Medical Association* **251**(5): 637–44.

5　Taroni F, Louis DZ and Yuen EJ (1993) Outcomes Management: The Italian Casemix Project. In *Diagnosis Related Groups in Europe: Uses and Perspectives* (eds M Casas and MM Wiley). Springer-Verlag, Berlin.

6　Gonella JS, Louis DZ, Zeleznik C *et al.* (1990) The Problem of Late Hospitalisation: a quality and cost issue. *Academic Medicine* **65**: 314–19.

7　Young WW, Swinkola RB and Zorn DM (1982) The Measurement of Hospital Casemix. *Medical Care* **20**: 501–12.

8　Neubauer G (1993) Germany: An outsider in DRG development. In *The migration of managerial innovation. Diagnosis related groups and health care administration in Western Europe* (eds JR Kimberly and G de Pourville). Jossey Bass, San Francisco.

9　Horn SD and Horn RA (1986) Reliability and Validity of the Severity of Illness Index. *Medical Care* **24(2)**: 159–78.

10　Horn SD and Sharkey PD (1983) *Op cit.*

11　Brewster AC, Karlin BG, Hyde LA *et al.* (1985) MedisGrps: A clinically based approach to classifying hospital patients at admission. *Inquiry* **22**: 377–87.

12　Hicks NR and Kammerling M (1993) The Relationship Between a Severity of Illness Indicator and Mortality and Length of Stay. *Health Trends* **25**: 65–8.

13　Oregon Health Services Commission (1991) Prioritisation of Health Services. *A Report to the Governor and Legislature.* Oregon Health Services Commission, Portland.

14　Bobadilla J-L, Cowley P, Musgrove P *et al.* (1994) Design, content and financing of an essential national package of health services. In *Global Comparative Assessments in the Health Sector* (eds CJL Murray and AD Lopez). WHO, Geneva.

15　Fung H, Chu YC, Chisholm K *et al.* (1996) *Patient Related Groups in Hong Kong. The Initial Experience.* Conference Proceedings Patient Classification Systems in Europe. Sydney, Australia.

16　Weiner J, Starfield B and Steinwachs D (1991) Development and application of a population oriented measure of ambulatory care case-mix. *Medical Care* **29**: 452–72.

17　Glover JA (1938) The Incidence of Tonsillectomy in Schoolchildren. *Proceedings Royal Society Medicine* **31**: 1219.

18　Kokkola K, Finell B and Lahdensuo A (1983) Regional Implementation of a Medical Care Programme in Northern Finland. *Community Medicine* **5**: 109–15.

19　Donaldson C (1995) Economics, public health and health care purchasing: reinventing the wheel? *Health Policy* **33**: 79–90.

20 General Register Office (1960) *Studies on Medical and Population Subjects No. 14.* Morbidity Statistics from General Practice. HMSO, London.

21 Boydell L, Grandidier H, Rafferty C *et al.* (1995) General Practice Data Retrieval: The Northern Ireland project. *Journal Epidemiology Community Health* **49(Suppl. 1)**: 22–5.

4   Mental health casemix development: where to and how quickly?

Introduction

The objective of casemix development activity in the arena of mental health, as in other health care domains, is the development of a comprehensive classification of needs, activities and outcomes for all mentally ill people receiving health and/or social care. Such a development would make a significant contribution to knowledge about, and management of, the mentally ill by health and social services. However, progress towards this objective is hampered by the separation of services between health and social care providers, and by the difficulty of collecting useful and usable information about the nature of health care interventions for those with a mental illness.

This chapter reviews work undertaken on classifications, casemix and minimum data sets applicable to service providers for the mentally ill and points the way for further work which is required if an acceptable measure of casemix usable with mental illness data is to be devised. It is not the intention of the chapter to review the litany of studies that have highlighted the difficulty of identifying variables that accurately predict resource consumption in this area, since this has already been done.[1-3] Work to date has been based on a general awareness of the considerable heterogeneity which psychiatric casemix groups commonly display and a search for factors that might reduce such variability.[4] Noticeably, the emphasis of the search has been on factors that tend to reflect aspects of the condition or status of the patient/client far more than on factors that reflect the interventions or regimen of care provided.[5]

The chapter therefore seeks to answer the following questions.

1 How much progress has been made towards the objective outlined, both in the UK and elsewhere, and what use can be made of the existing groupings?
2 Do the groupings, as presently constructed, have value for resource allocation or reimbursement, for internal resource management or other administrative purposes? (see Chapter 1)

3 What more should be done, or is being done, to secure progress towards
the objective outlined?

The argument for building a useful casemix measure to manage resources
in this area is, however, powerful. In the UK some 12% of the NHS budget
is allocated to these services (about £3 billion). Some 4498 hospital medical staff are occupied in caring for the mentally ill, accounting for more
than 200 000 inpatient admissions. These global figures (which exclude
community and social service activity) indicate the scale of governmental
resource associated with the care of the mentally ill compared with other
sectors. But they hide the range and emphases of expenditure within the
service. Table 4.1, recently compiled from burdens of disease,[6] shows the
relationship between spending on the mentally ill and spending on other
conditions.

Casemix classifications for the population with mental disorders and
the care and outcome of care for those populations would be useful, first
of all in offering a standard description and measurement of the types of
cases being referred, and the types of treatments being provided. Beyond
that, however, the challenge lies in making meaningful comparisons between
units dealing with the mentally ill, and then in adjusting reimbursement
for those units on the basis of real differences in need and resource use,
rather than on the basis of historical criteria.

The question of comparative analysis is raised by such data as are available. Figure 4.1 shows selected health districts (anonymized) in terms of
discharges with a diagnosis of mental illness. Cases and bed-days per thous-
and of the population vary dramatically between the districts. Again, it is
important to emphasize that the issue is not that there is no justification
for the differences, but that the absence of a clear and agreed approach to
measuring and comparing within this specialty area means that no discussion of the justifications for any differences can take place.

Mental health casemix and minimum data set specification

The dependence of casemix classifications on underlying data has already
been noted. Routinely collected person-based minimum data sets have been
defined and collected in mental health units for all inpatients for more
than ten years. However, the data have never been regarded as credible
within mental health services. Since basic data sets are such an essential

Table 4.1: Comparison of spending on the mentally ill with other conditions: 1992/93 estimated costs – NHS England; ranked by total expenditure

Disease group	Inpatient % expenditure of £12 144 m		Outpatient % expenditure of £2296 m		Primary care % expenditure of £3537 m		Pharmaceutical expenditure of £2059 m	
	%	£m	%	£m	%	£m	%	£m
Mental retardation	*6.91*	*839*	*0.26*	*6*	*0.00*	*–*	*0.00*	*–*
Stroke	5.55	674	0.32	7	1.47	52	?	–
Injury and poisoning	7.03	854	3.51	81	3.83	135	0.00	0
Mouth disease	0.31	38	0.62	14	25.95	918	0.00	–
Symptoms	4.05	492	8.69	199	5.74	203	0.00	–
Eye disorders	0.77	94	6.18	142	6.26	221	(0.5+0.8)	27
Dementia	*3.49*	*424*	*0.23*	*5*	*0.59*	*21*	*0.00*	*–*
Schizophrenia	*5.37*	*652*	*0.04*	*1*	*0.05*	*2*	*0.00*	*–*
Ischaemic heart disease	3.07	373	0.65	15	1.75	62	9.00	185
Other arthropathies	0.83	101	3.14	72	0.70	25	0.00	0
Normal delivery	2.99	363	5.76	132	0.25	9	0.00	–
Skin infections	1.69	205	5.28	121	2.96	104	2.20	45
Neuroses	*0.62*	*75*	*2.13*	*49*	*1.90*	*67*	*0.00*	*0*
Osteoarthritis	1.50	182	2.20	50	2.13	75	0.00	–
Rheumatism	0.66	80	3.29	76	1.15	41	0.00	0
Specific procedures and aftercare	3.06	372	0.00	–	0.00	–	0.00	–
Peptic ulcers	0.96	117	2.10	48	0.17	6	10.50	216
Asthma	0.60	73	0.50	11	1.42	50	11.00	226
Other non-organic psychoses	*2.42*	*294*	*0.53*	*12*	*0.45*	*16*	*0.00*	*–*
Other pregnancy	2.99	363	0.61	14	0.09	3	0.00	–

Source: *Burdens of Disease*: discussion document.
Mental ill health shown in italics.

prerequisite, this issue merits further exploration here. Three issues are important:

1 specification of appropriate items within the data set
2 collection of the data by all relevant personnel, and
3 accuracy and timeliness in data collection.

The first issue – specification of appropriate items within the data set – is clearly likely to be informed by a range of considerations relating to service provision and planning. The tripartite structure of needs, interventions and outcomes provides a useful approach to addressing this question. The following list is a basic set of data items.

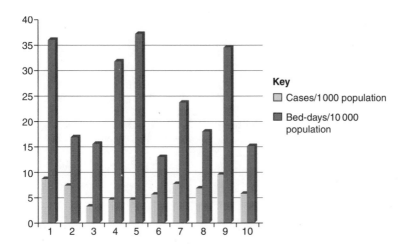

Figure 4.1: Selected health districts (anonymized) in terms of discharges with a mental illness.

- *Identifiers* (patient/client, treatment facility, primary care service responsible, payer)
- *Demographic elements* (address/postal code, date of birth, sex, ethnic status, marital status)
- *Condition/condition status* (symptoms, diagnoses, functional impairments)
- *Interventions* (treatment location/s, investigations/procedures, other interventions, medications, therapeutic approaches)
- *Legal status* (carer involvement/support)
- *Resources* (time spent by the services, time in hospital, location of contact or care: for example, inpatient, day hospital, outpatient or community-based care)
- *Outcome* (change in functional status, diagnoses, symptoms, time between discharge and subsequent re-admission).

The current emphasis on information collection in psychiatry has been more on needs (as expressed by symptoms or diagnostic information) than on interventions. Thus, little is known about the management of patients beyond their admission to hospital and the length of time they spend there. No data are currently collected about the treatment regimen or therapeutic strategy. Work to redress this is being put in hand, but it may be that one of the limitations in this area has been the dominance of the notion of 'procedure' from other areas of medical or surgical care. It is however important to acknowledge the reservations about measurement strategies, and concerns over the composition and use of routine data.

Table 4.2: Classification systems available for routine use by (psychiatric) health services

Dimension	Classification
Diagnoses	ICD 9, ICD 10, DSM III, READ*
Functional impairment	HoNOS (Health of the Nation Outcome Score)
Physical/functional/social disabilities	ICIDH (International Classification of Impairment, Disability and Handicap)
Social impairment	HoNOS
Needs	Mental Illness Needs Inventory (MINI)
Outcomes	HoNOS
Interventions, treatment	READ*

*Not strictly a classification.

Various of the items in the list on page 43 present problems in relation to their definition and interpretation. Emphasis on the collection of diagnostic information has not served mental health services well: assigning a psychiatric diagnosis is not always easy or consistently reliable. This leads to doubts about its validity, especially since the way in which the diagnostic classification is organized and described for mental illness is very different from other areas. ICD 10 recognizes 'the long-standing and notoriously difficult problems associated with the description and classification of (psychiatric) disorders ...'. The problems do not merely include the assigning of the correct psychiatric diagnosis but the difficulty of differentiating somatic conditions accurately. This means that there are patients with psychiatric conditions being classified as somatically ill. Wider knowledge and discussion of these problems would almost certainly improve the precision of the information being classified within a casemix measure.

The intention to collect information other than, or in addition to, the diagnosis has occasionally been discussed but only recently have significant efforts been made to introduce alternative coding and classification schemes which might reflect these areas. The available choice of classification systems for the areas identified remains limited (Table 4.2).

In psychiatry, perhaps more than in other disciplines, decisions about treatment are based on considerations about functional impairment at least as much as on the specific diagnosis. The use of information about aspects of functional status, social dysfunction and burden on carers could be considered as a routine element of mental health data systems, but this requires consideration of timing (when particular items should be collected) and of the process whereby such information is collected. Clearly, a model of 'remote' clinical coding is not viable if the record is based on clinically significant ratings which can only be collected in face-to-face interaction between clinician and patient.

How much progress has been made towards the objective?

The development of resource-based casemix measures in mental health has been trying to move away from a reliance on diagnosis as the main, or sole driver, of groupings to reflect resource consumption. Diagnosis Related Groups first utilized the ICD 9 diagnostic classification to define 25 DRGs covering mental illness and alcohol and drug abuse in two Major Diagnostic Categories. Use of the groupings within the prospective payment system in the USA was never seriously contemplated and a series of studies sought to identify more appropriate variables for casemix definition. Notwithstanding these studies and the dissatisfaction with the use of diagnosis as the sole measure, little in the way of new developments took place in the USA. Thus, Version 10 APR-DRGs utilizes an approach to defining psychiatric casemix which relies first in separating any occurrence of significant surgical procedure where a psychiatric diagnosis is present, followed by an allocation of records to groups based on a primary diagnosis. In these grouping schemes, as in other non-surgical areas, the diagnosis has been used as a means of categorizing the likely cost of a treatment episode.

Mental health casemix development in Australia, Canada, Sweden and in the UK has started to disentangle condition and activity dimensions. Australian work has been concentrating on an extension of patient-status variables, with research efforts directed towards assessing HoNOS items, a life skills profile and a clinician rated 'focus of care' item, which covers the treatment objective.[7] These measures are made on a two-weekly basis during the episode of care. Australia (within some states) has made greatest progress in starting some implementation of casemix-based reimbursement for mental health treatments using Australian national DRGs. Evidence of the impact of this move is likely to be important.

Swedish work has acknowledged that an understanding of treatment variables will assist in efforts to understand the resource implications of care. The development of SRGs (State Related Groups) has involved assessment of therapeutic inputs proposing the recording of up to six 'procedures' (covering a variety of medications and psychotherapeutic interventions), and information about parallel contacts.[8]

Work being undertaken within the mental health services in Israel represents an interesting development. The separate identification of therapeutic activities is being undertaken to provide a clearer view of the treatment. This can be compared with the characteristics of individuals receiving care.

The recording and use of treatment information is a significant element of work being taken forward within the English minimum data set and casemix development work. Proposals for a new mental health minimum data set are likely to provide for recording of information about therapeutic interventions, both with respect to pharmaceutical and psychological therapies being used. When added to status information it is likely that significant strides can be made in the definition of matrices reflecting needs, activities and outcomes for mental health services.

Research efforts that lay greater emphasis on patient attributes, such as diagnosis and functional status, improve the likelihood that measurement of outcomes will be practicable, within well-defined limitations, since the change in functional status is one of the most useful measures available.[9] However, such measures have correspondingly less value for the comparative assessment of resource usage for such patients. As this book argues elsewhere, it is clinical responses to patient states which account for resource use and measurement and classification of those which is therefore the key to this aspect of casemix development.

What practical use can be made of mental health groupings?

Diagnosis related groups for mental illness have a characteristically heterogeneous pattern when assessed against length of hospital stay or resource consumption. Reduction in variance statistics of between 6 and 15% (often depending on trimming of the data) reflect the lack of homogeneity relative to many other (especially surgically based) specialties. This heterogeneity has been the basis for consistent objections to any implementation of psychiatric casemix for purposes such as reimbursement or internal resource management. Development of groupings which include treatment variables should enable this difficulty to be overcome, since the costs of care will be more accurately described using such information.

There are however valuable uses for casemix in mental health, both of types of patient conditions and types of care package. These include their use in assessing needs and comparing rates of hospitalizations in order to consider issues of equity, access and availability of appropriate resources.

Second, simple outcomes can be assessed using existing groupings with HoNOS data to review functional improvements, or to review elapsed times between hospitalizations. Reimbursement linked to evidence of treatment success could have a significant influence on routine health provision.

Lastly, useful comparisons relating to simple performance questions can legitimately be raised through a casemix analysis of the costs of care. These should take the form of questions that are raised through the analysis which might lead on to further studies. It is important that they should not lead to hasty assumptions about inappropriate activity.

What remains to be done?

This chapter has argued that much work is necessary if real progress in understanding and measuring mental health provision is to be made. The work to be done includes the clear assignment of a diagnosis and the explicit and recordable structuring of treatments at the point of service delivery. Coding of these and analysis could provide useful information with which to establish, run and develop services. The relationship between costs, services and reimbursements could then be evaluated both locally and nationally. Such work would recognize that psychiatric services cover a range of sub-specialties, including services organized by age, acuteness or chronicity of the condition, as well as differing types of disability and need.

Work being undertaken in other countries has, if anything, more importance for mental health casemix development than for other areas, given the small numbers of developers and the complexity of some of the issues. Further reviewing and synthesis of such work needs to be pursued in order to ensure efficient development of useful groupings. In addition, evidence of the impact for mental health services of a casemix-based management approach would help to answer the question of how casemix developers, mental health administrators and policy makers can collaborate in developing and appropriately applying casemix tools.

References

1 Mcrone P (1994) Allocating Resources in Psychiatric Hospitals According to Casemix. *Psychiatric Bulletin* 18: 212–13.
2 Mcrone P and Phelan M (1994) Diagnosis and Length of Psychiatric Inpatient Stay. *Psychological Medicine* 24: 1025–30.

3 Creed F, Tomenson B, Anthony P *et al.* (1997) Predicting Length of Stay in Psychiatry. *Psychological Medicine* **27**: 1–5.

4 Oyebode F, Cumella S, Garden G *et al.* (1990) Diagnosis-Related Groups: Implications for psychiatry. *Psychiatric Bulletin* **14(1)**: 1–3.

5 Elphick M, Anthony P, Lines C *et al.* (1996) Mental Health Report: Casemix outcomes, resources, needs. NCMO, Winchester.

6 DHSS (1996) *Burdens of Disease*. October. (Cat. No. 96C0036). HMSO, London.

7 Mental Health Classification and Service Costs Project (1996) *Classification and Service Costs Project for Commonwealth*. Department of Health and Family Services. Shane Solomon & Associates.

8 Ivarsson B (1994) *SRG – State Related Groups*. SPRI Report 387. SPRI, Stockholm.

9 Avison WR and Speechley KN (1987) The Discharged Psychiatric Patient: A review of social, social psychological and psychiatric correlates of outcome. *American Journal Psychiatry* **144**: 10–18.

5   Healthcare Resource Groups and general practitioner purchasing

ROD SMITH, DAVID ARCHER AND FRAN BUTLER

Introduction

As the primary care-led NHS develops it is crucial that a sophisticated purchasing currency is developed to underpin it. Healthcare Resource Groups can be used as the purchasing currency to effect service agreements with defined casemix and at a clinical level to inform clinical practice, both in primary and secondary care. Because they can be used for large aggregated populations, such as primary care groups and whole health authority populations, they can be used to pick up subtle clinical information which would be missed at individual GP or practice level, such as longer lengths of stay in hospital than the national average.

Basic currencies

In the early days of the internal market contracts tended to be fairly simple. Finished consultant episodes (FCEs) priced at average specialty costs were just about adequate to support broad-brush block contracts. Counting tended to be incomplete and it was difficult to define whether increasing FCEs represented real volume changes or better counting. The efficiency index further confused the picture with perverse incentives to providers to overcount to 'increase their efficiency'.

Finished consultant episodes tended to be purchased at average specialty cost, all admissions within a specialty costing the same, i.e. a two-day asthma admission costing the same as a 364-day stroke admission. This was an unsatisfactory and crude purchasing currency which, because the casemix was not defined, carried considerable risk to purchaser and provider. A provider with limited financial resources could substitute 20 colectomies with 20 vasectomies, both in theory costing the same but in reality consuming hugely different resources.

A provider with average specialty prices was particularly at risk from a total purchasing group as they could withdraw work from the simpler end of the casemix, e.g. short asthma admissions outside hospital, leaving the complex end of the casemix in hospital, which would result in the hospital recouping only the average specialty cost for a more complex casemix.

The need for a more resource-sensitive purchasing currency

Fundholders' contracts have tended to be based on cost and volume, or cost per case and a crude casemix currency based on banded costing has developed (although with a wide regional variation).

It has become clear that a more sensitive purchasing currency is needed to ensure that resources truly follow patients. This becomes particularly important in the development of a primary care-led NHS. As services move out of hospital into the community, resources need to accompany the patients – earlier discharges and more day surgery require more community services.

It would clearly be impractical to price individually each episode of hospital care. There are already enough concerns about bureaucracy. By grouping together clinical treatments that consume approximately the same level of resources, a sensible purchasing currency can be developed which will support the agreements needed to develop the primary care-led NHS. Healthcare Resource Groups provide such a grouping.

The primary care-led NHS

As GPs and health authority purchasers get closer through total purchasing and commissioning groups, the potential to influence casemix increases. For example, some total purchasing groups have appointed discharge nurses to speed up (or sometimes slow down) discharge and help counter the widespread problem of delayed discharges. A service agreement based on average specialty cost would discourage this practice, even though it is beneficial to patients and the health service, because the resources needed for earlier hospital discharge would remain in the hospital and not be available to support the patient in the community.

More detailed pricing also allows comparisons to be made between different providers. This will in theory be most useful for purchasers in an area with a choice of providers, but also allows purchasers in the common position of having a monopoly provider to challenge the price and explore jointly with the provider ways of reducing the price. Detailed HRG pricing gives a direct focus on high cost areas on which to focus attention; these would be much more difficult to track down in an average specialty cost agreement.

An area that some GP commissioning groups (of whatever kind) will want to explore is the possibility of developing new types of provision. For example, respite care, which could be provided in an acute hospital, a community hospital, hospital-at-home or a nursing home. Prices based on average specialty cost would allow no rational economic judgement about which to choose, assuming that clinical quality of care was similar in all, whereas an agreement based on HRGs reflecting the actual cost in each of these settings could allow the most rational choices to be made.

Introducing HRGs into contracts

Change is always difficult and carries both threats and opportunities. The move from vague cost and volume contracts with ill-defined FCEs and average specialty cost to much more definable agreements based on casemix using HRGs carries risks to both parties, particularly during the transition period and needs to be handled with flexibility. However, an arrangement that rewards the provider with the correct resource for the work done and allows the purchaser to reduce resource consumption as casemix is changed is in the long-term interests of both parties. In areas where there is a competitive environment, sticking rigidly to average specialty costs will carry risks, particularly where other providers are shifting to HRG-based agreements. This is because purchasers, particularly true of GP-led ones, where the purchasers also make the referral decisions, could 'cherry pick' sending their more complex cases to the average specialty cost provider. In areas where there is a monopoly provider there may be a temptation to resist a move to HRG-based contracts, but in the long term it is in the provider's interest to let the simpler end of the casemix go and to work with a purchaser towards unblocking beds, shortening lengths of stay and shifting work into the community.

In Berkshire, the total purchasing group has moved most of its contract with the Royal Berkshire and Battle Hospital NHS Trust to differential pricing. For surgical specialties the prices are built up through HRGs and this is the purchasing currency, but for medical specialties, banded bed-day prices were used, rather than HRGs. For those specialties where prices are HRG-based, those FCEs with excessive length of stay (beyond the trim point, see below) move on to a price-per-day basis – this means there is an incentive to ensure that patients do not stay longer than appropriate, and GPs and other members of the primary health care team are well placed to question if a patient is ready to be discharged but remains in hospital.

In its first year the total purchasing group benefited from reduced costs as length of stay was shorter than the health authority average in most specialties. However, in neonatal paediatrics the move to day-bed pricing resulted in increased costs. We believe that the principle of paying the correct amount for the actual resource used is an important long-term principle, but the transition effects need to be handled flexibly and sensibly by both purchaser and provider recognizing that both share a common aim of using service agreements to improve the NHS for our shared patients.

Clinical improvement through HRGs

Although HRGs are primarily designed to provide groups of treatments which are of similar cost, they can also be used to increase understanding of comparative quality of care and outcome.

Patients who stay in hospital for longer than expected can be identified by using a trim point. This is defined nationally by the formula:

$$T = Q3 + 1.5(Q3 - Q1)$$

(T = HRG upper trim point in days; $Q1$ = lower quartile in days;
$Q3$ = upper quartile in days)

Approximately 7% of episodes nationally are longer than the trim point, although this varies by HRG. Patients remaining in hospital beyond this time are often known as 'bed-blockers'. This is a pejorative term and it is preferable to think of them as excess-resource consumers. That is exactly what they are doing and understanding why one provider unit has an excess of long-stay patients, and improving care once the problem has been recognized, can lead to better outcomes for the patient and reduce excessive resource utilization.

Case study 1: Discharge arrangements for fractured neck of femur

In the total purchasing project in Hemel Hempstead, 69 patients with HRG h36 (fractured neck of femur) were admitted to hospital during 1995/96, but only 55 of these patients (80%) were discharged before the national upper trim point of 47 days. Nationally, 95% of patients would be expected to be discharged by this point, so GPs, consultants and

Table 5.1:   Excess bed days by HRG

HRG	Trim point (days)	No. of patients	No. exceeding trim point	Excess (%)	Occupied bed-days	Excess bed-days
h38	47	69	14	20	2383	524
e35	16	91	12	13	825	96
e14	14	74	10	15	694	124

managers reviewed the notes of the 14 long-stay patients to determine the reasons for the extra hospital days, and the implications for the patients.

Although some of the patients were appropriately in hospital for longer than 47 days, a dialogue was set up and enabled change in the organization of discharge arrangements. Discussion with the trust regarding fractured neck of femur centred round the Audit Commission 1995 Report *United They Stand*. This gave an extremely clear and concise picture of the way coordinated care for elderly patients with hip fracture should be treated. The main recommendations were that the patients spent less than one hour in casualty, had prophylactic antibiotics and prophylactic thrombo-embolic prevention, had surgery with 24 hours and were rapidly mobilized, usually within 48 hours. The particular unit from which these data were extracted had problems with at least four of these five recommendations and we wait to see from the new consultants who have been appointed whether the Audit Commission's suggestions have been incorporated. Healthcare Resource Groups can be used for exception reporting in this way to identify 'black holes' of care, and to set up productive and informed dialogue. The national efficiency index is too insensitive to focus discussion, and merely sets up conflict between GPs and hospitals. It is far better for purchasers to ask providers to reduce by 3% the number of patients above the upper trim point in certain HRGs. This leads to sensitive purchasing, rather than the scatter-gun approach currently employed.

One obvious disadvantage of just looking at the trim points is that short lengths of stay do not necessarily indicate good quality care. If a provider has no patients beyond the trim point in, say, HRG e14 (myocardial infarction without complications), it may well be sensible to check that the reason is not that there is a high early mortality rate, before deciding to send all patients to that unit.

Case study 2: Organizing tertiary provision for angina

Using the example of e35 (angina >69) and e14, as well as h38, vast savings and improvement of care can occur as shown in Table 5.1.

The latter two examples are used because changes in purchasing policy occurred due to this information. The long-stay patients in HRG e35 (12 patients) and HRG e14 (ten patients) were reviewed and it was found that most were waiting for angiography or angioplasty at a tertiary centre and were awaiting a bed. By increasing the emergency contract for these procedures, better care to the patient was delivered and resources 'saved' from secondary provider (by reducing bed-days) were spent at the tertiary centre.

Case study 3: Analysing emergencies

Within the Berkshire Integrated Purchasing Project (BIPP), one of the objectives was to examine the rise in emergency admissions. Analysing the data using HRGs gave the project a better overall picture of which conditions were the most common and the level of resource used. As data become more accurate, particularly in total purchasing groups which are able to validate data within practices, annual comparisons become possible to look at how the casemix is changing. Although BIPP is a larger than average total purchasing pilot (TPP), with 89 000 patients, it is suspected that most of the changes can be explained by variation on small numbers. However, such comparisons can be a useful tool if a large change in the numbers of emergencies is experienced in order to focus on the areas of largest change. This will identify where discussions with the provider, or change of practice in primary care, is most likely to bear fruit.

Tables 5.2 and 5.3 demonstrate how the casemix has changed from one year to another.

Table 5.4 gives a general picture of the conditions and procedures for which patients are being admitted as emergencies, although it must be remembered that some HRGs are more specific than others and this will affect the number of FCEs that fall into each group.

The two conditions that proved of greatest interest in 1995/96 were 'sprains, strains and minor open wounds' and 'asthma and recurrent wheeze'. There was great interest from the GPs in the former category, as it seemed unlikely that such a large number of patients should be admitted in this category. A list of patients in this grouping was printed for each practice, but in most cases after further investigation the GP was happy that the admission was justified. Many of these were for head injuries (minor wounds of the scalp) where the patient was being kept in for observation. A similar exercise with asthma however showed that the management of some of the patients could be improved such that admission was unnecessary. In 1996/97 the number of FCEs covered by both of these HRGs has been reduced substantially compared to the previous year.

Table 5.2:   Comparison of non-elective FCEs by HRG, 1995/96 and 1996/97. Top 20 percentage decreases: non-elective FCEs

HRG	1995/96 Actual FCEs	1996/97 Actual FCEs	Difference FCEs	% difference	HRG description
s25	16	1	–15	–94	Rehabilitation
p34	24	11	–13	–54	Traumatic injury – paediatrics
p40	16	8	–8	–50	Congenital, other – paediatrics
p01	82	42	–40	–49	Asthma and recurrent wheeze – paediatrics
d13	15	8	–7	–47	Lobar pneumonia <75 without cc
h20	16	9	–7	–44	Non-inflammatory back and joint problems
m11	22	13	–9	–41	Major procedures uterus/ adnexae
p05	20	12	–8	–40	Obstructed airways (excluding asthma) – paediatrics
l36	15	9	–6	–40	Prostate disorders >74
s12	15	9	–6	–40	Other viral illness
d37	17	11	–6	–35	Other respiratory diagnoses >59 or with cc
l62	32	21	–11	–34	Miscellaneous kidney diseases, stones and trauma
p14	53	36	–17	–32	Other infections – paediatrics
l61	16	11	–5	–31	Kidney and urinary tract infections <70
h38	58	40	–18	–31	Neck of femur fracture >69 or with cc
h48	36	25	–11	–31	Sprains strains and minor open wounds >69 or with cc
p32	106	78	–28	–26	Gastrointestinal disorders – paediatrics
f06	19	14	–5	–26	Oesophagus >69
e13	20	15	–5	–25	Acute myocardial infarction with cardiovascular complications
d03	16	12	–4	–25	Chest procedures – category 2

Berkshire Integrated Purchasing Project/ Royal Berkshire and Battle Hospitals NHS Trust

Table 5.3: Comparison of non-elective FCEs by HRG, 1995/96 and 1996/97. Top 20 percentage increases: non-elective FCEs

HRG	1995/96 Actual FCEs	1996/97 Actual FCEs	Difference FCEs	% difference	HRG description
f37	7	21	14	200	Colon and rectum <70
d14	19	41	22	116	Bronchopneumonia >69
f16	10	20	10	100	Stomach and duodenum >69
f17	11	20	9	82	Stomach and duodenum <70
s01	11	19	8	73	Red blood cell disorders >74
e37	22	37	15	68	Chest pain >69
l53	9	15	6	67	Scrotum, testis and vas deferens disorders
j13	23	35	12	52	Cellulitis without cc
f35	12	17	5	42	Colon and rectum – category 2
e31	27	38	11	41	Arrhythmia and conduction disorders <70 without cc
f05	20	28	8	40	Oesophagus – category 2
p03	33	46	13	39	Upper respiratory tract infection – paediatrics
e32	17	23	6	35	Syncope and collapse >69
c07	33	44	11	33	Diagnoses category 1 >69 or with cc (mouth, head, neck, ears)
f65	15	20	5	33	Gastrointestinal bleed >69
p20	24	31	7	29	Seizures – paediatrics
h47	72	90	18	25	Closed upper limb fractures and dislocations <75 without cc
f47	71	86	15	21	General abdominal <60
e14	57	69	12	21	Acute myocardial infarction without cardiovascular complications
c08	36	43	7	19	Diagnoses category 1 < 70 without cc (mouth, head, neck, ears)

Berkshire Integrated Purchasing Project/Royal Berkshire and Battle Hospitals NHS Trust
HRGs are only included where there were 15 or more cases in either 1995/96 or 1996/97

Table 5.4: Thirty most common HRGs for non-elective work at the Royal Berkshire and Battle Hospitals (RBBH) Trust for the BIPP project

HRG	1996/97 Actual FCEs	Top 30 HRGs 1996/97 – BIPP/RBBH HRG description
m04	111	Minor procedures uterus/adnexae
h47	90	Closed upper limb fractures and dislocations <75 without cc
f47	86	General abdominal <60
p32	78	Gastrointestinal disorders – paediatrics
n11	73	Neonatal – high dependency
f84	70	Appendix – category 3
e14	69	Acute myocardial infarction without cardiovascular complications
e38	67	Chest pain <70
h49	65	Sprains strains and minor open wounds <70 without cc
a17	62	Non-transient stroke/cerebrovascular accident >59 or with cc
e44	56	Varicose veins
e19	55	Heart failure and shock
e35	53	Angina >69
e36	53	Angina <70
p04	51	Lower respiratory tract infection – paediatrics
n09	48	Neonatal – low dependency
h43	48	Closed pelvis and lower limb fractures and dislocations <70 without cc
p03	46	Upper respiratory tract infection – paediatrics
c07	44	Diagnoses category 1 >69 or with cc (mouth, head, neck, ears)
c08	43	Diagnoses category 1 <70 without cc (mouth, head, neck, ears)
p01	42	Asthma and recurrent wheeze – paediatrics
d39	42	Other respiratory diseases
s15	41	Poisoning toxic effects and overdoses <65
d14	41	Bronchopneumonia >69
h38	40	Neck of femur fracture >69 or with cc
e31	38	Arrhythmia and conduction disorders <70 without cc
e37	37	Chest pain >69
p14	36	Other infections – paediatrics
n05	35	Neonatal – other
e29	35	Arrhythmia and conduction disorders >29

Conclusions

The case studies described previously show some of the potential uses of casemix analysis from a general practice purchasing perspective. Other work which could be undertaken includes:

• comparison of the rate of neonatal admissions per 1000 births compared to the health authority purchaser rate
• further examination of the appropriateness of admission and the effect of possible preventative measures for the most common HRGs
• further comparison of rates of HRGs for the TPP population compared to those for other local purchaser populations.

In order to undertake these sorts of studies it is necessary to have some basic resources. These include the ability to provide costs, and undertake analyses.

Costing

Some providers will be more keen than others to provide costs/prices for separate HRGs. However, providers are expected to use HRGs to underpin their pricing mechanisms in particular specialties, and producing prices for HRGs may not be a difficult further step in other specialties. A major consideration is that the monitoring of contracts or agreements where there are large numbers of separate prices can be time-consuming for the provider and the purchaser, and needs to be fully automated if it is to be feasible.

The information provided by such monitoring is however extremely valuable, as the spend on each HRG is then clearly identified, pointing to where efforts might be directed if spend is to be reduced.

Analysis

The analyses described above by Hemel Hempstead and Berkshire do not require any complex statistical methods. Minimum data sets (MDSs) for the population and time period in question are required and these can be processed through the grouper available from the National Casemix Office (NCMO). For the Berkshire project, MDSs supplied by RBBH already contain the HRG as an additional field. Using the basic spreadsheet skills available in most practices, it is possible to analyse length of stay, determining the percentage of patients with length of stay exceeding the trim point, and the HRGs which account for the greatest number of episodes.

Also using basic spreadsheet skills it is possible to list out those patients covered by a particular HRG, or those whose length of stay exceeds the trim point, and patient notes (in primary care, secondary care or both) can then be examined for those patients as described above. Expert information analysis skills are not needed.

Summary

General practitioners in total purchasing projects and commissioning groups are in an ideal position to pursue detailed work using HRGs, because they can focus on individual patients falling into each group, and can discuss with consultants the reasons for any exceptions highlighted by pricing or analysis at this level. The purpose of using HRGs in this way is to encourage friendly, informed and positive debate with clinicians, not to settle scores with hospitals. The use of HRGs as a tool to help purchasers look in the right place and ask the right questions helps to move the development of primary care-led purchasing forward by focusing on the resources used by the patient, and by pointing to areas where clinical discussions with the provider would lead to change in practice and better and more efficient care for patients.

6   Case study: Costing, contracting and resource management

ALAN BUTLER, JEREMY HORGAN AND LISA MACFARLANE

Introduction

This chapter describes how the costing for contracting methodology has been developed and applied in a busy University Hospitals Trust and how practical approaches to resource management using casemix have been put into place.

Following the introduction of the NHS internal market, heralded by the 1989 White Paper *Working for Patients*,[1] Southampton University Hospitals Trust realized that average specialty costing would not provide a sufficiently sensitive currency to cover variations in case type and case complexity. Average costs could be skewed by high-cost procedures and, if they were then used for contracting, all purchasers would pay the same price for very different services. Local purchasers, for example, could be paying for district general hospital-type services at specialist prices. The trust was vulnerable on two fronts – either in underpricing expensive services by averaging costs down or in setting uncompetitive rates for routine care to cover high-cost procedures – a more sensitive measure was needed and HRGs seemed to provide the answer.

It was therefore decided to undertake crude casemix costing for the first year of contracting so that prices reflected real resources used – money needed to follow the patient for the hospital to remain competitive and to recoup appropriate costs from the right purchasers.

The need to develop more sensitive contracting currencies added impetus to earlier resource management initiatives – in particular it acted as a catalyst for bringing together information in the trust about patients, resources (staff and facilities) and costs, and for analysing the relationships between them.

Setting and managing directorate budgets

Southampton University Hospitals Trust has a strong clinical directorate structure covering groups of specialties who are responsible for managing a devolved budget and subsequently for securing income from contracts. Budgets were initially allocated to directorates and support departments on the basis of workload and staffing in a way that still ensured total hospital expenditure was subject to overall control. From an organizational point of view this was sensible, as fluctuations across directorates would in all probability balance each other out. While it is essential that directorates have responsibility for balancing devolved budgets and incentives to become and remain efficient, financial control across the organization as a whole has to be maintained. This means that while clinical directors have control over the purse strings in their directorate, it is also acknowledged that they are part of a bigger picture and have the difficulty of balancing devolved responsibility while ensuring corporate accountability.

Expenditure within the Trust is made up of variable activity related costs, semi-fixed and fixed costs including capital charges. These costs are allocated either to clinical directorates who control direct expenditure or central directorates who control overheads. These are brought together in contract prices that reflect the total costs of providing health care with overhead apportionment ensuring that total 'corporate' expenditure is covered. While this shares the burden of overhead costs, just like block contracts based on average costs, it provides little direct incentive to clinical directorates to save indirect costs other than through a corporate sense of responsibility and goodwill. The challenge then is how to move traditionally-based budgets towards a more directly managed accounting model at directorate level based on the service being provided, the level of expenditure and in turn, contract income. It also poses the question of what measure of activity – currently finished consultant episodes – is appropriate to achieve that and how best to reflect the costs of a differing casemix. Healthcare Resource Groups offered a manageable common currency to define casemix and similar-cost procedures.

Applying costing methods at a local level

In 1993, the NHS Steering Group on Costing[2] issued guidance on how to price contracts. Importantly, it stressed the principle that price should as closely as possible reflect cost but this posed problems at a time when costing systems had not been developed to examine resources below specialty-level. A methodology was developed across Southampton University Hospitals Trust to produce a set of prices based on HRGs that could be

Table 6.1: HRG-costed specialties

Group 1 – 1994 for 1995/96
- Orthopaedics
- Gynaecology
- Ophthalmology

Group 2 – 1995 for 1996/97
- General surgery
- Urology
- Vascular surgery
- Neurosurgery
- ENT
- Oral surgery

Group 3 – 1996 for 1997/98
- Cardiac surgery
- Paediatric surgery
- Paediatric orthopaedics

used for setting casemix-sensitive contracts which would ensure that all costs could be recouped. In parallel, a very detailed activity-based costing project in the Wessex Neurological Centre set out to identify key cost drivers and potential cost-weights to improve the sensitivity of prices and help refine HRGs.[3]

With the introduction of the purchaser–provider split, the trust recognized the importance of allowing for the effects of casemix when setting contracts. As a large teaching hospital (1500 beds across 50 specialties), including a number of specialist services as well as the usual local services, the mix of health care that is provided to our non-host purchasers is very different from the service we provide to our host purchaser and GPs. This is true at the specialty and sub-specialty levels.

Initially, we used local groupings of procedures, based for example, on DRGs, or BUPA classifications as well as earlier versions of the HRGs. Mandatory costing of HRGs was welcomed because it provided a nationally agreed and understood method of grouping activities and standardized our whole approach.

During 1994/95, 1995/96 and 1996/97 all surgical specialties were costed (Table 6.1) using the methodology outlined in the *Guidance on Costing for Contracting*.[2]

A common methodology was used, dividing the process into four distinct stages (see Figure 6.1).

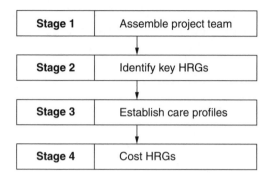

Figure 6.1:   HRG costing process.

Stage 1: Assembling the project team

Each specialty had a project team which met fortnightly over a period of about four months, and typically comprised:

- a consultant from the specialty
- a second consultant, or member of the junior medical staff
- a ward nurse
- a theatre nurse
- the information officer
- the directorate accountant
- the clinical service manager
- a costing accountant.

Stage 2: Identifying key HRGs

Key HRGs which represented over 70% of the costs incurred and/or the bed-days occupied within a directorate were identified. The reporting software provided by the National Casemix Office (NCMO) was used to analyse a complete year's data; for example, in neurosurgery this identified eight HRGs that required detailed costing and the numbers of each procedure that had been grouped to those key HRGs. The 70% rule was then applied to the procedures to select those requiring care profiling. These data were then shared with the project team for the specialty concerned to agree which HRGs and which procedures within those HRGs would act as the basis for directorate contracts.

The first task of the team was to examine the analysed data. The depth and length of the discussion varied from specialty to specialty and depended on the quality of the data and how far the HRG analysis coincided with the teams' perceptions of their main activities. There was of course a level of error in the data, for example uncoded and unclassifiable episodes, but this was in general less than 5% and was not felt to affect the overall picture significantly.

This scrutiny also highlighted the distorting effect that some outliers can have. For example in ENT there was a particular episode with a three-month length of stay that clearly distorted the average for that HRG and also its rank in the analysis by bed-day. By using national trim points, extraordinary outliers could be extracted; episodes just outside the trim points were retained in some instances where their lengths of stay were only a day or so in excess of a relatively short average length of stay for the HRG. This level of outlier is a predictable proportion of activity and as such part of the normal activity of the trust.

When the team was satisfied with the data, agreement was reached on the key HRGs and procedures. Where HRGs contained procedures of relatively low volume but high cost these were included in the list of key procedures. For example, the final list of key HRGs for neurosurgery was extended from eight to ten.

Stage 3: Establishing care profiles

Project teams proceeded to draw up care profiles which identified the level of resources being typically consumed for key procedures within each HRG. Care profiles identified:

- average length of stay
- time in theatre
- total consultant time
- total junior medical staff time
- prosthesis cost
- pathology tests
- radiology examinations
- significant drugs and consumables cost
- number of nursing dependency days.

Based on available data, assumptions were made about each resource grouping: for instance only drugs and consumables of a significant cost or quantity were identified – there was no attempt to identify every last aspirin or swab used.

For ward-related nursing costs, rather than use length of stay as a method for apportioning costs, the individual days of the episode were weighted for the 'usual' level of dependency. The levels ranged from one to four; four being the most dependent and one the least dependent. Typically, the day following the procedure was the most dependent day and the day before discharge the least dependent. Even where data were not being recorded, the nurses seemed to have little difficulty in determining a 'likely' dependency of the typical patient. This approach was found to have a significant effect on the relative costs between HRGs and, although crude, was nonetheless felt to reflect the resources used more accurately.

Individual members of the team were tasked with completing different sections of the care profile according to their expertise. This multidisciplinary approach worked well in both splitting the job into manageable tasks and creating a sense of common ownership.

Stage 4: Costing the HRGs

The subsequent care profiles then had standard costs applied to them derived either from the direct costs of the specialty or average costs for support and overhead departments. Relative costs did not always match clinicians' preconceptions or what the structure of the HRGs might imply, so in these cases the profiles were amended if required after investigation and final care profiles were then agreed.

Using cost information in contract pricing

The trust costing development team used the costs derived from this exercise to set base contracts as a starting point for negotiating in the following year. The trust had derived a 'quantum of cost' for the coming year which reflected the level of expenditure expected to be incurred for the anticipated level of activity. This total cost was then split between specialties using allocation and apportionment methods. All clinically related costs from overhead departments and support services were passed down to the level of the specialty providing the service for which income could be generated and added to the direct costs identified in that particular specialty budget. This process is in itself a very large task which falls outside the scope of this chapter.

Each specialty then had an identified 'expected' cost with a matching target level of activity. This target activity was split into a casemix using the previous year's HRG analysis. Given the specialty total, the target casemix and the costs derived from the HRG exercise, projected costs by HRG were calculated for the coming year.

These projected costs were applied to the target casemix analysed by purchaser. This resulted in a base contract for each purchaser that had a total for each specialty based on projected cost and, underlying it, an assumed casemix. We had therefore recalculated the contracts using the actual

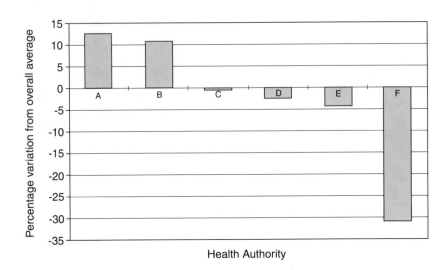

Figure 6.2:   Variation in contract prices to reflect expected casemix.

casemix from the previous year, the HRG costs from the exercise uplifted for increases to our base costs, and a revised target for each purchaser:

Number and type × Cost per = Contract income by purchaser
        of HRGs   HRG

At this point each of our purchasers had a contract based on the same tariff. However, their average specialty costs for the same specialty might be widely different and this was because we had taken into account the different casemix of each purchaser and applied appropriate costs to that casemix.

For example, Figure 6.2 shows the percentage variation in average specialty cost for neurosurgery between different purchasers. The host purchaser is significantly below the overall average cost for the specialty, with the two other main purchasers of the service being significantly above. If no allowance had been made for casemix then our host would be substantially overcharged for the service and the other two purchasers significantly undercharged. A similar chart could be produced for each of our specialist services which would show the same sort of variation to a greater or lesser degree.

Neurosurgery is a key service for the trust with a very high average cost per episode. The trust has therefore developed contracts for this service to reflect the variations in casemix, both between purchasers and within year. Contracts are drawn up not with an underlying casemix assumption, as in other specialties, but with an explicit stated target activity for each of the key HRGs. This is monitored on a quarterly basis and extra income is generated or refunds made to each purchaser depending on the variation by HRG from target.

For the other specialties where HRG costing has taken place, the assumed casemix is re-based each year using the latest actual figures available. Casemix shifts are therefore reflected but in a delayed fashion. It is hoped to develop in-year monitoring of shifts in casemix from the expected level. While probably not moving towards the cost and volume contracts used in neurosurgery, the information will be used instead to shadow-monitor the contracts during the year and raise significant variations in contract review meetings. Work is now under way in this area.

Initial contract proposals apply the same tariffs to all purchasers. However, as contract negotiations progress, and for example marginal costs are negotiated for increases in target activity, the tariff rates for individual purchasers drift from the original base and will be significantly different between individual purchasers if allowed to 'drift' over a period of years. The re-basing of contracts annually on a common tariff prevents this variation in price becoming excessively distorting.

The original tariffs derived from the exercise are used to set both the GP fundholder (GPFH) and extra-contractual referral (ECR) tariffs. There are however differences between the two; for example trimmed bed-days are excluded from the costs in the ECR tariff but included in the GPFH tariff because there is no mechanism for collecting the trimmed bed-day cost from GPFH and probably limited benefits in doing so.

Work is also taking place to compare our tariffs with other providers – a task that was made very difficult in the past by a lack of a common costing currency, even though the overall methodology is expected to be the same. The proposal to compile a national database of all HRG costs is therefore very welcome.

Internal management of activity based on casemix information

In-year shifts in casemix can now be accounted for, albeit with a built-in delay, but constraints or ceilings still exist on the amount of extra work that will be bought. Contracts may indeed be significantly reduced in subsequent years if caseload drops. Either can have an impact on the effective use of resources through over- or undercapacity and subsequently affect the costs of providing care – referrals therefore have to be controlled to ensure:

• targets are at least met but not excessively exceeded

- available resources are maximized and, most importantly
- the patients in most need can be treated and treated when they need it most.

So how do casemix-based contracts help internal resource management? The need for more sensitive contracting currencies has prompted detailed investigation into the processes of care, in particular the way activities related to different types of patients impact on costs. A detailed study within the Wessex Neurological Centre using barcode technology[4] illustrated how HRGs with a similar overall cost (or price) use internal resources in very different ways – some were heavy users of ward nurses, others had a high impact on theatre or intensive therapy unit (ITU) staff, for example. This is not necessarily important to know for price setting, but is crucial in judging how best to manage resources at a directorate level. Whereas the cost of care may be similar for two different patients, the way care is provided may be very different: the quality of care that can be provided may also vary depending on the casemix and severity of casemix within a ward at the time. Profiles of care for each professional group have therefore been identified so that a degree of prediction is now possible about the likely 'burden' on nursing staff, the impact on ITU beds, the requirement for theatre, magnetic resonance imaging (MRI) or computerized tomography (CT) scanning facilities. This in turn allows better planning of waiting-list admissions, staff rosters or allocation of staff to shifts, for example.

Shifts in caseload (and hence shifts in costs) can be picked up quickly and trends identified: more importantly, the reasons behind changes in activity levels can be more readily explained in a clinically relevant way:

- who is referring more/less (of what)?
- has the epidemiology changed for that condition?
- are (certain types of) day cases increasing because of a new technique?
- likewise is length of stay falling?
- what is the readmission rate for that condition?
- are specialist referrals increasing to a particular consultant?

Once activity is identifiable by the patient's condition, treatment and costs of care, it becomes possible to make informed judgements about how to manage change – both operationally and strategically.

Resource management remains a fine balancing act between clinical priority, capacity to treat and cost. In Southampton an attempt is being made to bring these three together by building a decision support system to model relationships. This will allow operational decisions to be more responsive to the needs of individual patients and create the flexibility required to alter work patterns in response to changing contract specifications.

Conclusions

The trust has reached a stage of consolidation in costing, where the contracting methodology is being refined rather than replaced and the emphasis has shifted to using existing costing information to reap in-year benefits in terms of income recovery, casemix monitoring and budget setting.

Looking two or three years ahead, the areas for development will be the medical specialties where the allowance for casemix at the moment in contracts is crude or non-existent. It will also encourage purchasers to take more account of casemix data when making purchasing decisions. For example, targeting high-volume low-cost procedures of limited benefit and high-cost low-volume procedures causing cost pressures to the trust.

Resource management has become a practical reality now that sufficiently detailed data are routinely available to support everyday decisions about quality and quantity. With ever-improving integration of information technology, coupled with the development of increasingly sophisticated analytical and data interpretation skills at directorate level, operational decision-making and strategic planning can be truly 'informed'. While professional judgement will and should always play a part in setting priorities, resource management as a process can help disentangle whose judgement and whose priorities. Finally, it can enable a move away from simple efficiency drives to more comprehensive measures of clinical effectiveness.

Costing at the level below specialty is very important for hospitals with a varied casemix. HRGs allow the use of both a nationally accepted grouping methodology and implementation programme to enable the Trust to contract and receive income on a realistic basis and to internally manage resources more effectively.

References

1 DOH (1990) *Working for Patients*. Department of Health (Cmnd 555) HMSO, London.
2 National Steering Group on Costing (1994) Guidance on Costing for Contracting. NHS IMG, Leeds.
3 Connel N, Connell N, Lees D *et al*. (1996) Costing and Contracting in the NHS: A Decision Support Approach. In *Management Accounting in Healthcare* (eds M Bourn and C Sutcliffe). CIMA Publishing, London. pp. 29–40.
4 Lees P and Macfarlane L (1997) Barred Facts. *Health Service Journal* 107(5544): 26–9.

7   Performance management and audit

NIGEL WOODCOCK AND KEN LLOYD

Introduction

In our rapidly changing NHS there is a critical need for communication. In particular, effective communication requires that everyone speaks and understands a common language covering the clinical care which we provide for our local populations. This must offer grouping of clinical activity at a level of aggregation which is suitable for use by clinical teams, local management, and the wider planning and prioritization of health care spending. We believe that Healthcare Resource Groups (HRGs) now go a considerable way to providing that language.

Northampton General Hospital NHS Trust was involved in the development of HRGs from their inception and has used the expertise developed locally to put them to practical use throughout many areas of trust management at clinical department level. Internally to compare the relative performance of different clinical services, and externally to compare the performance of clinical services within the trust against those of similar organizations.

For the first time since the introduction of the internal market, finance staff have the tool to bring them an appreciation of the complexity of the issues surrounding clinical management and an understanding of the frustrations so often felt by clinical staff when resources are not available to them.

Equally, many clinical staff are now able to appreciate the financial constraints facing management at trust level and are able to put their expertise and energy into formulating a better way forward.

Another benefit provided by HRGs is that information produced can be used to identify the areas with potential for clinical audit and to highlight the need for the development of clinical guidelines and/or care pathways. Not only does this fulfil the primary purpose of enhancing patient care but provides health commissioners and purchasers with hard evidence of a 'value for money' service.

Our aim has been to introduce to all clinical specialties across the trust the full potential of using HRGs and to work with them to develop a practical and useful clinical management system. To achieve this we needed to show that HRGs are not just a 'costing for contracting' currency but a powerful tool which is able to provide busy clinicians and clinical managers with answers in their continuing drive to improve the quality and efficiency of patient care.

Background

Clinical activity relates to and informs the commissioning process and in an area of the country facing tough financial decisions and substantial increases for demand for both elective and emergency care, there has been a need for commissioners and providers to have valid, mutually comparative information available to inform the contracting process.

For the trust, this was used not just externally with the commissioners, but it was also required for use internally, at every level from clinical team to board level.

In addition to HRGs informing the contracting process, we felt that the quantity and mix of cases anticipated and hence the expected consumption of resources by specialty would be necessary in the development of clinical services for the future. This was likely to be required, whatever the method of funding, and on the basis of this we felt that we could develop realistic specialty-based budget requirements for future years.

In the event we found that although there was a considerable amount of work required for data collection and analysis the value of the information to the trust made this justified. As an example, comparisons of the shapes of the length of stay distribution and the overall mean were useful in examining what resource usage would be expected from current performance and used as a benchmark for future clinical activity.

Analysis of these distributions also provided source information on which to base clinical audit and, most importantly, where to focus our interest and to prioritize further work.

Methodology

An analysis of the requirements for providing casemix information within a number of key specialties was undertaken. It was agreed that if HRGs were to be useful to clinicians and managers, then the information produced needed to be instantly available to all relevant staff, both clinical and managerial, up to date, and easily understood. This required the implementation of a front-end package to the casemix system which provided executive information reporting.

Our starting point in this development was to address a number of key issues.

- 'Data gathering' within the trust, focusing on both the recording and physical flow of activity data and how this could be improved.
- The assessment and monitoring of data quality in order to provide data that were consistently reliable. Previous attempts within the NHS to develop care or even to describe the status quo through analysis of clinical activity have been difficult because of poor quality data with low credibility.
- Development of clinical resource profiles for identified HRGs which can assist in the development of the profile of cost for all the elements of care and cost contributing to the individual HRG. This was of necessity a complex process involving many staff and sources of information but again crucial to the credibility of the exercise.
- Topic focused clinical audit in which a particular topic area, for example hip replacement, and all the associated treatments/processes are reviewed with a variety of audit methodologies to assess the outcomes of treatment and patient care.
- Computer aided analysis of HRG data to help interpret casemix data. Even though 'casemix systems' have been available to clinical services for many years and a great deal of clinical and financial information has been fed into them, in many places, there have not been suitable analytical tools to help clinicians use and understand the data. At Northampton much of the work necessary to achieve this step in the evolution of casemix analysis was done 'in house'.
- Delivering HRG information reports to the clinical directorates. The need for the developments outlined was well recognized within the trust and developing the specialty-based reports was given priority. Dealing with the information however required considerable maturity of approach from all sides and a fair compromise between providing absolute confidentiality and open publication of results to stimulate change.

As mentioned above, the analysis of data gathering within the trust highlighted the need to address data quality. Clinical coders were reorganized to work with clinical teams on ward rounds to produce the most meaningful coded clinical data for input into the casemix system. This was seen to be a major step forward in achieving the goal of accurate and trusted information. It was also vital to endorse the importance of clinical coders and their work to the trust as a whole. Whereas clinical coding had previously been a neglected area, it was now important for all those involved with patient care to understand that contributing to accurate clinical coding is a necessary element of clinical practice. Quite literally, the viability of a specialty or indeed the whole trust might depend on producing an accurate reflection of clinical work undertaken.

The development of clinical resource profiles enabled clinical staff to specify the resources required for any one particular HRG and gave them the major input into the costing of clinical services. This not only improved the accuracy of the clinical input into costing but also developed working relationships between clinical and finance staff. The clinical resource profiles were designed to provide information on the significant resources used, for example:

- inpatient/day cases
- theatre usage (including pre-med. and recovery)
- implants
- high cost drugs and consumables
- wards (including nursing skill mix)
- other diagnostic and treatment support
- any other high cost items.

Trust-wide analysis

Using the national hospital episodes statistics (HES) data as a benchmark, the current clinical performance and relative efficiency of a large number of clinical specialties were assessed (Figure 7.1). We were reassured that in the majority of specialties, performance against available casemix-sensitive benchmarks was very good.

Taking trust performance as a whole it was clear that we were already more 'efficient' in the accepted sense than would be expected taking into account our casemix and range of specialties.

It is particularly important to note at this point that without a casemix weighted analysis, a trust such as ours – carrying out a more extensive range of services, and more complex procedures than an average District General Hospital – would typically only appear to be of average efficiency or even be spuriously criticized for poor performance.

Analysis across a range of specialties allowed us to take stock of our priorities for action in a way that had not previously been possible. Comparative information showed that some clinical areas – where we had previously felt concerned about the pressure of work and availability of beds and resources in general – were indeed performing very efficiently. In

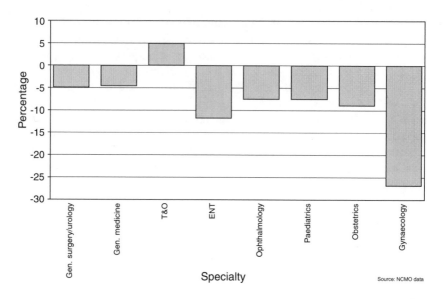

Figure 7.1: Percentage difference between NGH and expected mean length of stay (LoS).

these areas we gave priority to service developments and staffing adjustments aimed at alleviating strain.

It was also clear from a clinical management point of view that it would be unrealistic to plan for growth in activity in such areas without adding resources, primarily in the shape of key staff and dedicated beds and facilities.

In discussions with commissioners, this accurate benchmarking of current performance allowed for much more realistic discussion. In simple terms we knew where we could stoutly defend our performance and decline to offer them an efficiency gain – and equally where we could help them respond to extra demands for care by improving our productivity.

Demonstrating to commissioners clinical areas where we were seeing substantial changes in casemix year on year also helped in prioritization of funding and in the avoidance of mutually unsatisfactory 'bottlenecks' in the provision of care.

Another feature not previously practical was the ability to demonstrate, through casemix-weighted information, that an apparently unchanged level of activity in strictly numerical finished consultant episode terms within a specialty could conceal marked changes in the profile of resource use and associated costs.

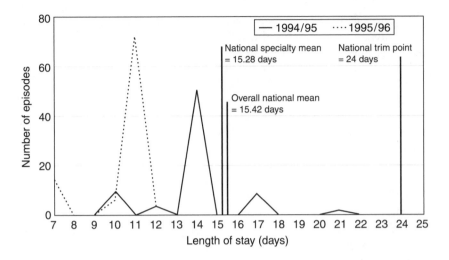

Figure 7.2: Specialty: orthopaedics. Length of stay distribution: HRG – h01 – primary hip & replacement (exc. knee).

The information provided by the computer aided analysis of HRG length of stay distributions led to topic-focused clinical audit in several areas – particularly where we felt there might, on further analysis, be grounds for discussing changes in clinical practice.

Hip replacement

The orthopaedic specialty and, as an example, HRG – h01 – Primary Hip Replacement was one of these identified groups (Figure 7.2). A series of audits was designed to address patient care during an inpatient episode for primary hip replacement. These included:

- admissions policy
- total hip replacement operative procedure
- physiotherapy
- wound infection total hip
- replacement/revision
- discharge policy.

For 1994/95, it was clear that although most patients were discharged by 14 days, which was less than the national average, there were a number who were staying for longer periods, and this affected the mean length of stay locally in this specialty.

Recommendations from the audits included the introduction of several care plans and pathways and the reorganization of care to provide post-discharge nursing support in the community. In l995/96 the orthopaedic activity was again grouped into HRGs (see Figure 7.2). The plot of h01 clearly shows the reduction in patient length of stay and reduced numbers of patients staying longer than the average. Patient readmission rates and complications during inpatient stay were analysed to see if there was any reduction in quality of care, and happily there was none.

Concurrent with the clinical audit programme a pilot OutReach scheme was introduced for patients undergoing hip replacement. The NORTH (Northampton OutReach to Home) project was run by the orthopaedic department with support from the general practitioner core group. Thirty patients were selected for the scheme according to medical and social criteria. The outcomes sought were a quality service as measured by patient, carer and professionals and a demonstrable reduction in post-operative length of stay in hospital. Clinical audit of the pilot scheme indicated the following.

- The average length of stay for the 30 patients on NORTH was 7.4 days.
- Average home stay after ward discharge was 4.6 days.
- There was a saving of 130 bed-days during the six-month project period which led to an increased bed occupancy and reduction in the waiting lists.
- NORTH patients required on average 4.2 home visits.
- An audit of primary care teams, patients and carers was undertaken with the following results:
    84% of GPs did not think their workload had increased
    70% of GPs considered the scheme to be good
    100% of patients said they were confident about being at home and satisfied with their care
    100% of carers were happy for the patient to be included in NORTH.
- Complication rates, as measured by re-admission or infections were less than those experienced by non-NORTH patients. It must be remembered however that patient numbers included in the pilot scheme were small.

Stroke

Stroke is an important cause of death and an even more significant factor in disability and health costs. Over a two-year period, 411 patients were admitted to Northampton General Hospital (NGH) with a diagnostic HRG grouping for stroke. At present, stroke cannot be cured but can be prevented and there are opportunities to alleviate disability and handicap.

To have an impact on behaviour change, the 'target audience' should particularly be receptive to change and the message should be delivered in a timely manner by a credible source of information in a clinically relevant way. In collaboration with GPs and the Northamptonshire Health Authority a set of clinical audits was designed to review the care of patients admitted to NGH with a diagnosis of stroke. The objective was two-fold:

1 to review treatment and diagnostic procedures and to introduce standard indicators of care for hospital management
2 to establish clinical guidelines for primary care, secondary care and rehabilitation on the overall management of these patients.

Since the introduction of the stroke guidelines stroke admissions have decreased by some 25%. Obviously this is encouraging but more work still needs to be done in the area of stroke prevention/management.

Oral surgery

Information on the total number of episodes, either aggregated for the hospital or on an individual specialty, defined by HRG, can be used to determine apparent activity changes at the level of aggregation illustrated by casemix. These changes explain many of the reasons for either an underspend or overspend of budget within a clinical area. Changes in casemix also highlight areas where contracts need to be reassessed either by adjustment of resources within the existing contract or in extreme instances a renegotiation of the contract. Figure 7.3 highlights such a casemix change in oral surgery. The reasons behind the change, and the implications for patient services obviously need to be addressed by both clinicians and managers within the specialty.

Analysis of the change indicated a more complex casemix which was attributable to the appointment of a consultant with an expertise in facial reconstruction work. The result of the change was a decrease in extra-contractual referrals (ECRs) for the purchasing authority and an increased budget deficit for oral surgery. Healthcare Resource Group evidence of casemix highlighting the change was used to re-negotiate the oral surgery contract with the purchaser to reflect the reversal of ECRs.

Conclusions

Casemix analysis of activity and performance using HRGs has become the backbone of the trust's monitoring procedures, allowing a range of staff

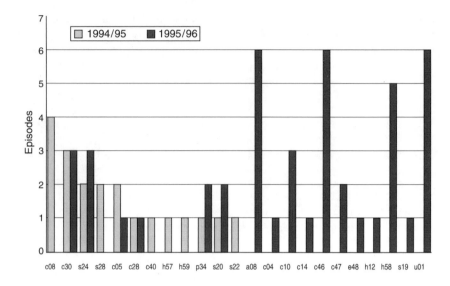

Figure 7.3: Oral surgery HRGs (excluding c16, c15, c26, c06) for 1994/95, compared with 1995/96.

c08 – Diagnosis category 1 <70 w/o cc

c30 – Skin and bone procedures category 3 w/o cc

s24 – Planned procedure not carried out

s28 – Other admissions <65

c05 – Mouth and throat procedures category 1 w cc

c28 – Diagnoses category 3 <70 w/o cc

c40 – Skin and bone procedures category 4 w/o cc

h57 – Extracranial procedures for trauma – category A

h59 – Removal of fixation device

p34 – Traumatic injury

s20 – Complications of treatment <55 w/o cc

s22 – Convalescent and relief care >49 or w cc

a08 – Other nervous system procedures

c04 – Nose procedures category 1 w/o cc

c10 – Skin and bone procedures category 1 <65 w/o cc

c14 – Nose procedures category 2 w/o cc

c46 – Mouth and throat procedures category 5 w/o cc

c47 – Skin and bone procedures category 5 >69 or w cc

e48 – Amputations – major

h12 – Soft tissue and other bone procedures – category A <70 w/o cc

h58 – Extracranial procedures for trauma – category B

s19 – Complications of treatment >54 or w cc

u01 – Ungroupable

groups to understand and participate in improving the quality and efficiency of services.

Analysis of HRG-weighted performance by specialties against the peer group has also enabled the trust to have confidence in its clinical strategy and has informed and shaped negotiations with health commissioners and the contracting process. Healthcare Resource Group profiles for length of stay are being used widely throughout Northampton General Hospital to identify areas such as h01 where, with the help of clinical audit, clinical management can be modified to improve patient care whilst reducing length of stay.

Development of HRGs as a management and clinical audit tool has provided many benefits. Principally these are seen to be:

- a 'common language' for purchasers and providers
- patients receive the best possible health care available within available resources
- casemix reporting is more informed by the use of HRGs
- health commissioners/purchasers can focus on some outcome data to show they are buying a 'value for money' service
- future services are planned more accurately using reliable information
- clinical staff are more aware of the need and importance of accurately recording diagnoses/procedures/drugs and the damage that poor data could do to patient care.

Finally, it is worth adding the caution that although we have found HRGs to be a very valuable aid to clinical management, there is clearly a great deal more to do, and greater potential in the use of HRGs in the future. Healthcare Resource Groups do not currently cover the whole spectrum of work carried out even by hospital-based services, this must be recognized and taken into account so as not to limit the validity of analyses. When data sets and groupings are available across the spectrum of care, it should be possible to provide a more accurate picture of the total package of care received by patients.

8   Case study: Use of casemix to support purchasing in Doncaster

DAVID MEECHAN

Introduction

The purpose of the NHS is to secure through the resources available the greatest possible improvement in the physical and mental health of the people of England.[1] Within this overall purpose, NHS purchasers (health authorities and Primary Care Groups/Trusts) have the responsibility of assessing the health needs of the local population and securing services which are both clinically effective and represent a good use of taxpayers' money.

This chapter describes how casemix measures are being used by Doncaster Health Authority to help ensure that it achieves the greatest possible health gain from the resources available for the 300 000 people for whom it has responsibility. Casemix measures are being used in two main ways. First, in order to make sure that the value of the contract with its main acute provider, Doncaster Royal Infirmary and Montagu Hospital, reflects fairly the complexity of workload undertaken. Doncaster Health Authority should thereby achieve value for money by paying a price which is more closely related to the cost of providing the treatment.

Second, comparative data are being used in order to benchmark provider performance to identify areas where there might be scope for efficiency gains or improved outcomes and to assess the appropriateness of levels of activity purchased.

Use of casemix to calculate contract values

Background

Since the introduction of the NHS 'internal market' inpatient contracts between health authorities and hospitals have typically been of the cost and volume type. With this approach the contract value is based on an expected number of finished consultant episodes (FCEs) in each specialty. The contract value is then usually adjusted to reflect differences between actual activity levels and this baseline, often using marginal specialty costs.

Table 8.1: Weighted activity: 500 FCEs of each of type A and type B

Casemix group	Cost weight	FCEs	Weighted activity (FCEs × cost weight)
Type A	10	500	5000
Type B	1	500	500
		1000	5500

However, there are risks to both the provider and purchaser with these cost and volume contracts where activity is measured only at the specialty level. A more complex casemix than expected may mean that, in order to achieve agreed activity levels, the provider's costs exceed contracted income. On the other hand, a shift towards a less complex casemix than expected may lead the purchaser to expect extra activity or a reduction in the contract price in order to obtain 'value for money'.

In 1993, a joint research project was initiated by Doncaster Health Authority and Doncaster Royal Infirmary (DRI) and Montagu NHS Trust to examine how casemix measures could be used to monitor acute inpatient contracts. The project received financial support from Trent RHA.

The aim of the project was to develop a methodology for monitoring contracts and calculating contract values which reflect actual workload undertaken more sensitively than do FCEs at the specialty level. The objective was to use a measure of activity which is weighted for the complexity of the casemix treated, so that a major procedure could contribute more than a minor one.

However, it was felt that it was not appropriate to move to cost per case contracts at individual procedure level as this would require too much administrative effort.

A simple example

The concept of weighted activity can be illustrated by a simple hypothetical example. Assume that a specialty contains only two types of case, type A and type B, where type A is a major procedure that costs ten times more than the minor procedure type B. Also assume that the expected contract activity is 500 FCEs each of type A and type B. This gives an expected (baseline) weighted activity of 5500 as shown in Table 8.1.

Now suppose that what actually happens under the contract is that only 400 FCEs of type A are treated and 600 FCEs of type B. This means that the total number of FCEs for the specialty (1000) is exactly as expected.

Table 8.2: Weighted activity: 400 FCEs of type A and 600 FCEs of type B

Casemix group	Cost weight	FCEs	Weighted activity (FCEs × cost weight)
Type A	10	400	4000
Type B	1	600	600
		1000	4600

However, the weighted activity is 16% below target (4600 against an expected of 5500), calculated as shown in Table 8.2.

So, in this example, the use of casemix weighted activity would result in an under-performance against contract and a lower contract value than if total specialty FCEs had been used.

Research project

In moving from the theory as described in the above example to a practical way of monitoring contracts, the following questions had to be answered by the research project.

Which casemix group should be used?

First of all it was decided that it was not appropriate to develop local groupings. It was felt that this would require too much effort and would not offer any opportunity for comparative analysis.

At that time there were two main classification systems that were in use in the UK; DRGs and HRGs. It was agreed that both DRGs and HRGs would be used to monitor contracts in 1993/94. In fact, the results were similar using both classification systems. Given the subsequent development of HRGs and their use in the 'costing for contracting' initiative, it was decided to drop DRGs in future years and use HRGs.

How should cost weights be calculated?

Initially, the Finance Directorate at DRI derived cost weightings for each HRG based on average length of stay with adjustments to reflect the relative use of operating theatre time. For HRGs with a small number of cases, regional average lengths of stay were used instead. As more accurate HRG costs became available through the 'costing for contracting' exercise, these were used.

How should baseline activity be calculated?

Baseline activity for each HRG was based on the previous year's contract activity. Cases covered by GP fundholding and which related to practices which were to become new fundholders were excluded to give an expected profile for activity under the DHA contract. This profile was then applied to the contract activity level in each specialty to give the baseline casemix.

Adjustments were made to this baseline to reflect any known changes in casemix, for example the development of a new endoscopy unit.

Attempts were also made to adjust the baseline for the casemix of patients on the waiting list. However, difficulties with assigning patients to casemix groups and forecasting future waiting list trends meant that this was not possible.

So far, no attempts have been made to influence prospectively the casemix baseline to reflect, for example, desired changes towards more effective treatments.

What are the implications for information systems and clinical coding?

In order to support this use of casemix to monitor contracts, both provider and purchaser information systems needed enhancing. The DRI needed to add the HRG to contract minimum data sets and to produce contract monitoring reports comparing actual and expected activity by HRG.

Doncaster Health Authority was successful in obtaining funds from the NHS Executive's 'Developing Information Systems for Purchasers' (DISP) programme to enable its contract management system to integrate with the HRG grouper and to provide automatic monitoring of HRG based contracts.

Clearly, this method of contracting is dependent on accurate and complete clinical coding, as without this a case cannot be assigned to its appropriate HRG. Therefore, additional resources were put in to improve the timeliness of coding.

How should contract values be calculated?

It was agreed that contract values would be calculated using the same principles regarding floors, ceilings, tolerances and marginal costs to weighted activity as had previously been applied to FCEs.

Project roll-out

This method of monitoring contracts was piloted during 1993/94 and has been rolled out as follows.

- *1993/94* Casemix used on a shadow basis (i.e. no financial adjustments made) for gynaecology, ophthalmology and general medicine.
- *1994/95* Contract value based on the HRG mix for the above three specialties.
- *1995/96* Contract value based on the HRG mix for the above three specialties and also oral surgery. Also contracts for ENT, orthopaedics and urology monitored on a shadow basis HRG.
- *1996/97* Contract values based on the HRG mix for the above seven specialties and also general surgery.

Some results

Elective ophthalmology

Figure 8.1 shows the relative cost weights that were used in 1995/96 for the six most common ophthalmic HRGs. The cost weights are based on local lengths of stay, theatre costs and significant implants and disposables.

It can be seen that in general the cost weights increase from HRG b01 to b06 reflecting the increasing resource consumption of the conditions treated. These range from minor procedures in b01 through to cataracts in b04 and b05 to complex procedures and corneal grafting in b06.

Figure 8.2 compares the actual and contract (expected) activity in 1995/96 for elective ophthalmology for each HRG.

It can be seen that there were fewer cases than expected in the lower cost HRGs (b01 to b04) but significantly more than the contract baseline in b05.

So, although the overall number of FCEs was close to the contract target, there had been a shift towards a more complex casemix, which resulted in a small additional payment over the base contract value.

In fact, the reason for the shift was a change in clinical practice to use phakoemulsification to remove the cataracts. This procedure aids rapid visual recovery, reduces the risk of postoperative problems and costs more because it depends on high technology equipment and an expensive folding plastic lens. The phakoemulsification procedure groups to the more resource-intensive HRG, b05, rather than b04 which is where cataract procedures were previously assigned.

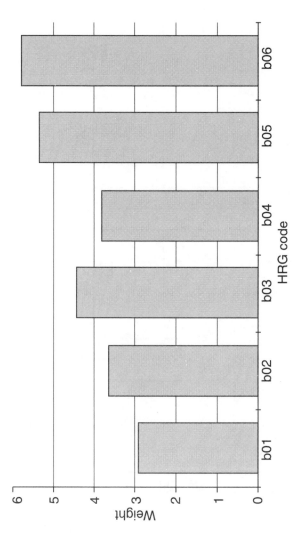

Figure 8.1: Elective ophthalmology weights 1995/96.

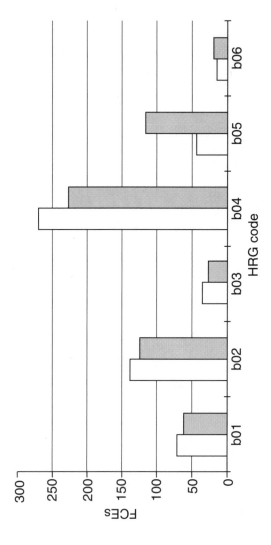

Figure 8.2: Elective ophthalmology activity 1995/96.

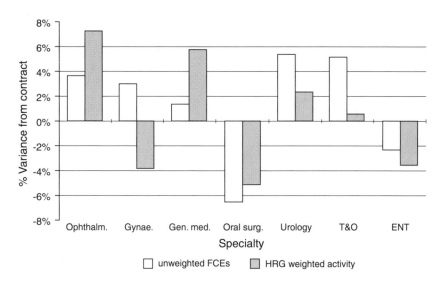

Figure 8.3: The effect of HRG weighting on contract performance (full year 1995/96).

Effect of HRG weighting on contract performance

The effect of using HRGs to monitor contracts in 1995/96 is shown in Figure 8.3.

The graph compares for each specialty the variation against contract in terms of both unweighted FCEs and HRG weighted activity.

It can be seen that, as has been discussed previously, ophthalmology FCEs were 3.7% above contract but, because of the shift towards a more complex casemix, weighted activity is 7.3% above. General medicine and oral surgery also show a more complex casemix. On the other hand, gynae-cology, urology, orthopaedics and ENT show shifts towards a less complex casemix than expected.

The aggregate effect over these specialties was that the contract value was approximately £30 000 more than it would have been on an un-weighted FCE basis.

General medicine non-elective

Figure 8.3 shows that the general medicine casemix was more complex than expected, giving an HRG weighted activity variance of 5.8% above contract, whereas unweighted FCEs were only 1.4% above.

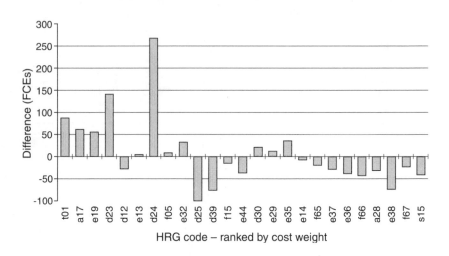

Figure 8.4: Difference between actual and expected activity: general medicine and geriatrics non-elective 1995/96.

The reason for this shift is shown in Figure 8.4. The graph shows the difference between the actual and expected number of FCEs for each of the top 25 HRGs ranked by cost weight (highest cost HRG on the left, lowest on the right).

It can be seen clearly that there was an increase in the number of high-cost HRGs such as t01 (dementia) and d23 and d24 (chronic obstructive airways disease) with a decrease in low-cost HRGs such as s15 (overdoses) and e38 (chest pain).

The reduction in the number of low-cost HRGs can be explained by the setting up of a new medical assessment unit, the aim of which is to prevent avoidable admissions. It is likely that those patients for whom admission is avoided fall into the low-cost HRGs (e.g. conditions that require a period of observation and signs and symptoms which do not result in more serious diagnosis).

Purchaser issues

Accuracy and completeness of clinical coding

As with this method contract payment depends on casemix, it is important that the clinical coding is accurate so that any apparent changes in case-mix are real rather than artificial. The ability to audit coding is therefore important in order to avoid a situation similar to that of 'DRG creep', experienced in the USA whereby cases are incorrectly coded so that they are assigned to a higher cost category.

Efficiency index

The NHS Executive measures health authorities' performances in meeting efficiency gain targets using the 'efficiency index'. As this efficiency index gives equal weight to all inpatients and day cases, it does not take casemix into account. Therefore, if the casemix becomes more complex, the method of contracting described here will have an adverse effect on the efficiency index (expenditure would increase more than activity). Conversely, a less complex casemix would improve the efficiency index.

Limitation of FCEs

Because HRGs are assigned to FCEs, this method still suffers from the inherent limitations of FCEs as a measure of activity. For example, every time a patient is transferred between hospital consultants, or is re-admitted, a new FCE is generated. Therefore, it is important that the rates of transfer between consultants and re-admission rates are also monitored.

Financial risk

This method of contract payment potentially adds to the financial risk for the purchaser if the casemix becomes more complex. Therefore, a ceiling was agreed which limits the financial adjustment which can be made because of casemix shifts.

Comparative casemix information for benchmarking

Provider performance

The role of health authorities and Primary Care Groups/Trusts as purchasers of health care includes ensuring that services provided represent value for money. In an ideal world this would be assessed by comparing the costs of treatment between different providers. However, although costing information is improving through the costing for contracting initiative, accurate comparative costs are not currently available.

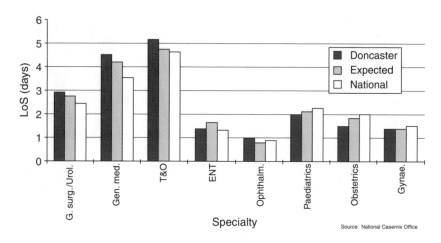

Figure 8.5: 1994/95 National and Doncaster Health Authority mean LoS, with expected mean LoS for eight main specialties.

Hospital lengths of stay and day case rates are alternative indicators of efficiency which are commonly used. However, it is often claimed that comparisons are not 'fair' because 'our casemix is different'. Indeed, it is true that a hospital with proportionately more complex cases would be expected to have longer lengths of stay and lower day case rates than a hospital with a less complex casemix.

Therefore, it is important that comparisons are adjusted for differences in casemix. Figure 8.5 compares the average length of stay (LoS) for activity purchased by Doncaster Health Authority in 1994/95 with both the national average and the expected LoS. The expected LoS is what would be expected if the national average had been achieved locally for each HRG.

It can be seen that in general surgery/urology, for example, Doncaster's average length of stay is about 0.4 days above the national average. However, the expected LoS is significantly higher than the national average, indicating that Doncaster has a more complex casemix. The fact that Doncaster's LoS is only about 0.1 days above the expected level shows that, *having adjusted for casemix*, local performance gives less cause for concern.

Figure 8.5 also shows that Doncaster's LoS is higher than expected in general surgery/urology, general medicine, trauma and orthopaedics and ophthalmology and lower than expected in ENT, paediatrics and obstetrics, with gynaecology almost equal to the expected level.

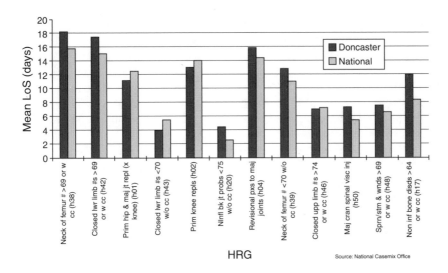

Figure 8.6: Doncaster Health Authority, trauma & orthopaedics: top 12 HRGs (by bed-days), mean and national mean LoS 1994/95.

Similar comparisons on day case rates have also been used to identify specialties where local performance is below the national average, after allowing for differences in casemix.

These top-level indicators have then been used as a basis for discussion with the main local acute provider to identify areas where there might be scope for efficiency gains.

For example, Figure 8.5 suggests that Doncaster has an above average LoS for trauma and orthopaedics. This has been investigated further by comparing the local LoS with the national average for each of the top 12 HRGs. It can be seen from Figure 8.6 that the LoS for the HRG which uses the greatest number of bed-days, h38 (neck of femur fracture aged over 69 or with complications or co-morbidities), is more than two days above the national average.

This type of information, and more detailed information at procedure level, is now being used by the local hospital in discussions with its clinicians to identify how LoSs might be reduced without adversely affecting the quality of care provided.

Although standardizing for casemix using national average HRG values undoubtedly makes comparisons significantly more meaningful, there are inevitably factors other than those relating to relative efficiency which might explain differences from the norm. For example, Figure 8.5 shows that

Doncaster's LoS for general medicine is above the expected level. However, locally there is no activity coded to the specialty of geriatric medicine as all elderly medical inpatients are included within the general medicine specialty. It would therefore be expected that Doncaster's general medicine LoS for HRG a17 (Stroke/CVA aged over 59) would be longer than the national average, as nationally much of the longer stay activity within this HRG relating to elderly patients will be recorded under the geriatrics specialty heading.

Therefore, it is important that casemix-adjusted comparisons are used as indicators which inform discussions and raise questions requiring further investigation rather than as providing answers in their own right.

Effectiveness and outcomes

As well as comparing provider performance in terms of LoS and day case rates, Doncaster Health Authority is also using routine data to assess effectiveness and outcomes. This includes comparing local performance both over time and against external benchmarks on a range of indicators including:

- readmission rates
- hospitalization rates for procedures where cost-effectiveness has been questioned (e.g. D&C in women aged under 40, insertion of grommets, etc.)
- death rates within 28 days of elective surgery
- cancer survival rates
- GP practice referral rates.

This information is being used in discussions with local providers and GPs to identify areas where there might be scope for improvement and to agree local action plans. For example, following a study comparing readmission rates, the local hospital has agreed to undertake a detailed audit of readmissions in one specialty where readmissions appeared to be relatively high.

It is important that the assessment of effectiveness using comparisons between areas and over time is sensitive to differences in casemix.

Conclusion

This chapter has described two ways in which casemix measures are being used by Doncaster Health Authority to help it to achieve the greatest possible health gain from available resources.

First, it has been shown how HRGs are being used to achieve value for money from local acute contracts by ensuring that contract values reflect the complexity of the casemix treated.

Second, the use of casemix measures to compare provider performance and to assess effectiveness has been described.

Comparisons against benchmarks based on accurate information which is sensitive to casemix provide a useful starting point for local discussions. Such discussions can identify areas where there is scope for improving efficiency and effectiveness and should lead to agreed action plans.

The development of a primary care-led NHS is giving increased influence to GPs in the purchasing of health care. Therefore, it is important that primary care purchasers are aware of the benefits that casemix information can offer and that casemix developments are responsive to the needs of primary care. A project is currently under way in Doncaster with a total purchasing pilot group of practices to identify their information needs and to assess how to gain maximum benefit from such information.

The development of HBGs should help in this process by improving the understanding of the relationship between patients' conditions, treatments and outcomes.

Reference

1   NHS Executive (1996) *Priorities and Planning Guidance for the NHS.* Department of Health, Leeds.

9 Clinical management and measurement

TIM SCOTT

Introduction

This chapter looks at the role of the clinical director, with particular reference to clinical directors in acute hospitals, and considers the use of aggregated information to support the management role. In particular the fundamental need to look comprehensively at clinical workload and identify specific 'clusters' of work suggests application of HRGs.

Getting started as a clinical manager

How do you get on to a moving merry-go-round?

Many clinical managers describe their initial experiences of management as 'being thrown in at the deep end'; 'jumping on a moving bus' or 'getting on a moving merry-go-round'. At first glance the above question might sound entirely hypothetical, but perhaps there is relevant experience to consider.

A trip to Disney World with a cautious, intelligent, analytic four-year-old ('Actually, I am nearly five!') provides some insight. For a start there is always a queue for the rides. Far from being a boring and irritating necessity, this is a chance to discuss what lies ahead, seek clues as to the experience and, particularly, look at the faces of other people who have just finished the ride. 'Is there going to be a fast bit?', 'Will I be scared?', 'Will you hold my hand if I am frightened?'. The child endeavours to build up a picture of the likely experience ahead and draw in the resources around, be they friends or relatives.

In many peoples' pocket will be a well-thumbed and dog-eared copy of *Birnbaum*, the official guide to Disney. Faced with the enormity of Disney World some families read up on the various rides to see what they want to do and also to get some understanding of what the ride is like. 'Is this a very bumpy ride?', some will want to know. So a little research helps.

As you get nearer to the ride itself you see smiling attendants helping people on and off. These experienced professionals clearly know exactly how to get on and tell you just how to do it – and anyway you are able to watch the people just in front of you. Finally we are safely aboard. 'No, I'll sit in the middle and you sit on one side and you sit on the other.' Often that first ride is conducted in almost complete silence – the child intensely absorbing the experiences and storing them for later discussion and analysis. Things move so fast there is no time to comment on something or worry about something before the next bump is ahead of us. Finally, after a physically and emotionally enervating series of highs and lows we draw towards the exit. Again the professionals ensure that people move on to the moving pavement and out of the cars and we watch intently how the people in front manage – often trying to do it better than they did. And, after a successful and enjoyable ride the usual response is 'I want to do that again now!'. Sometimes, if one member of the family has not yet gone on the ride they will be cast in the role of neophyte to be taught by the experienced; 'Come on, I am going to take you on a ride and show you how it is done!'.

Of course the metaphor is not comprehensive or exact. In particular, the participant in a Disney ride is essentially passive, whereas a clinical manager is (hopefully) active and participates in the whole experience. Nevertheless, there are a number of insights to be gained about structuring and tackling the role. The obvious and unsurprising revelation is the need for some understanding of the role and some clarification of expectations, as well as perhaps some training, prior to taking up the role. Clinical managers do need to talk to colleagues, preferably from other locations, about their experience in the role and what it has entailed. You need to know what might happen and what will happen and you can only explore this by talking to a reasonably wide range of individuals. 'What is the job like if the trust gets involved in a merger?', might be an area worth exploring, for example.

Consideration of the Disney experience might lead trust executives and others to think a little bit more about succession planning. The whole business of getting on and off is a lot easier if the ride has been properly designed, for example if there is a moving walkway just beside the embarking and disembarking area. Do the professional managers act like the attendants at Disney, easing clinical staff into management roles and ensuring confidence? How well designed is the induction training for the clinical director post? To what extent, if any, is any consideration given to people leaving the post, to help them move back into other roles, whilst still drawing on the experience that they have gained?

Researching the role

Some background reading on clinical directors and the clinical directorate role should help. There are probably around 4000 clinical directors (or clinical leads, clinical co-ordinators or clinical managers) in NHS trusts in the UK. The range of different roles and positions is quite startling but, as with any statistically normal distribution, for most clinical directors the jobs are relatively similar. The typical, or modal, clinical director is likely to be 45–49 years old, and directly accountable to the chief executive for their management role. Most will command a budget of some £2–3 million, and are expected to provide a managerial lead for some ten consultant colleagues. The average time spent on managerial issues is over four sessions – in general more than their contract specifies – with numbers of support staff unlikely to rise above two. Fortunately, most will have a job description, although a significant minority do not, and it is likely that the average clinical director finds their management responsibilities cause problems in fulfilling their clinical role.

Most clinical directors will receive some development or training which they consider to be very helpful during their time in the job – but most identify time management and budget analysis as areas for further skill training, along with dealing with complex change and difficult colleagues as areas for further management training. Significantly, the vast majority hold no formal management qualification. Most are rewarded financially for their managerial work and receive one or two additional sessions. However, it is also likely that they will feel undervalued for their managerial contribution, and it is an issue of concern that many trusts regularly hold meetings of the executive team without clinical directors.

Research on the role of clinical director has dispelled a number of the early myths. As with medical directors, the full range of consultant specialties is represented, in roughly the same proportion as the general consultant body (Figure 9.1). It is not a pre-retirement job and the age range is only a few years older than the general consultant age range (Figure 9.2). (The above description is drawn from research by BAMM.[1])

The starting position

In Disney the wise child marshals and organizes their support well in advance of the ride and checks the degree of experience in the group as a whole. They need to know, in an emergency, who they will cling on to and

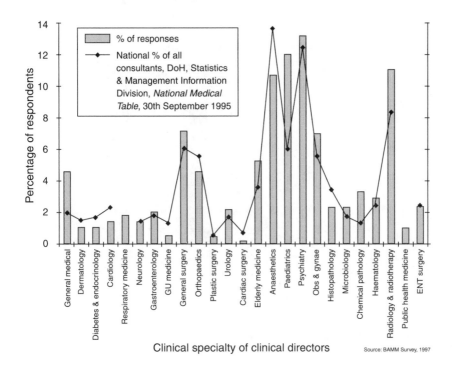

Figure 9.1:   Range of clinical director specialties.

that this is acceptable. Similarly, the clinical director will want to discuss in advance the support available from colleagues and also acquaint themselves with their direct support team. When the gale blows and you are shouting 'Head for the North East!', it is nice to know that the person at the helm is an experienced business manager. The immediate management task that faces newly appointed clinical directors varies not only according to their experience, preparatory training and other qualities, but also according to the directorate itself and its immediate prior histories. A range of possibilities is set out in Figure 9.3.

The boxes give some indication of their likely applicability – the higher the percentage, the more likely the scenario. One would imagine that any directorate that was well established and well running would have established some induction process and be part of a larger organization with a commitment to helping you get on and off the merry-go-round. Regrettably, few clinical directors are likely to find themselves in the bottom

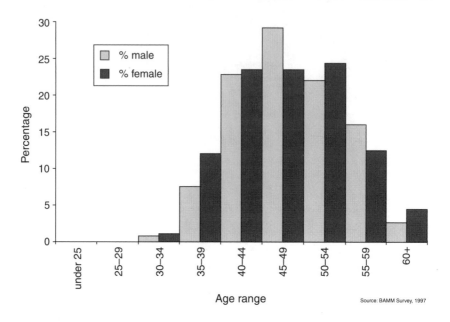

Figure 9.2:   Age range of clinical directors.

righthand corner box – that is trained and inducted comprehensively to take over the management of focused and well-running directorates. It should, of course, be one of the objectives clinical directors set themselves, to hand over in this way, in due course, to a colleague.

The immediate management task

Whatever the experience or preparedness of the clinical director, their initial management approach will be largely driven by the circumstances in which they find themselves. Faced with a directorate which has not been actively managed, the first imperative must be to get a grip on the basics of day-to-day management.

Most clinical directors anticipate a need to start with people, particularly consultant colleagues. 'It's all about managing people isn't it?'. Well, yes and no. No clinical director can function without at least passive support and approval from consultant colleagues. Any individual consultant can, if they choose, severely disrupt the directorate and its work. This kind of

	No induction or training	Quick handover and some training	Comprehensive induction and handover and substantial prior training
Little prior active management of directorates – a mess	60%	30%	10%
Basic operational management in place but little sense of shared purpose	25%	50%	25%
Smooth running, well managed with clear identity and sense of purpose	15%	20%	65%

Figure 9.3:   Newly appointed clinical director.

open warfare, although rare, does sometimes break out and is intensely destructive and often very difficult genuinely to resolve and heal. It is of course to be avoided at all costs and it is important that clinical directors establish a good working relationship with other consultants. One definition of management is 'Keeping the people who have made up their minds about you separate from those who are still willing to give you a chance!'.

It would be a foolish clinical director who neglected the other clinical professionals – particularly nurses. Initial reactions to clinical directors in many trusts in the early 1990s were concerns by nursing staff at 'Being managed by a doctor'. To a very large extent these have disappeared as clinical directors have made it clear that what is important is their clinical directorate and that they hold no special brief for medical staff. Nevertheless, some mistrust persists and it will be important visibly and consciously to address the concerns of senior nursing staff and establish dialogue with them. However, all of this, whilst absolutely and fundamentally necessary to smooth-running directorates, is in no sense sufficient to ensure the management of the directorate.

Direction and momentum

The clinical director needs to have a very clear picture in their mind of what the directorate is attempting to achieve and the resources with which it is hoping to achieve it. Aspects of this will be found within the budget and also within the operational plan, assuming that these exist, and in the first instance, understanding these and discussing the issue of delivering them is the immediate management task. Of course, the broader question is, 'Are these appropriate targets and objectives and appropriate resources?', but the clinical director will need to tackle the management of the current situation before attempting to introduce change.

In the typical patient care directorate, such as general medicine, general surgery or obstetrics, the prime resource is people. Clinical directors may not need to know precise numbers of staff; typically there will be some 200 full-time equivalent staff working in the directorate. What most clinical directors will look at is some kind of breakdown of staffing into specific functional, or geographical, areas. 'There are three staffed 18-bed wards and seven staffed outpatient clinics a week.' The numbers linked to each of these service points will no doubt be a matter for discussion and debate, as to whether staffing is at the right level, but the total number of, say nursing staff, in the directorate is, in itself, relatively meaningless.

Initially the clinical director will be concerned about the current momentum of the directorate. Is it broadly on target, failing to deliver the required level of service, failing to live within resources or, worst of all, failing on both of these counts? A quick stock take, as well as discussions with the chief executive, medical director and business manager, should soon establish the immediate position and give some indication of the time available to achieve results. If it is six months into the financial year already and the budget is currently projected to show a 5% overspend at the end of the year, then there are only a few weeks to cut back on expenditure and live within budget. Similarly, if the directorate is significantly understaffed with vacancies not covered by locums or agency staff, then the lead time to actually getting new staff in post is likely to be two or three months and again suggests the need for urgent action.

> 'I need some information'
>
> 'What sort of information?'
>
> 'Well, what sorts have you got?'
>
> 'Lots of different types, what do you need?'
>
> 'I'm not sure, but I know I need some information'
>
> Adapted from Welch N (1993) Informed decision making. *British Journal of Health Computing*
> **10**: 15–17.

Figure 9.4: 'Needing information ...'.

Finance and budgets

Having established the immediate managerial position the clinical director will want to work with the business manager and with the (nominated) management accountant from the finance section to look at all aspects of the budget. There will almost certainly be some uncertainties about income, with possibilities of monies for special projects, special work, inflationary pressures and so on. The clinical director will need to get a clear picture of the sums involved and the likelihood of their realization. There will also be areas of the budget not directly linked to staff salaries and the possibilities for reducing costs. Whilst the focus of management, particularly the Chief Executive Officer and Director of Finance will be on the over- (or under-) spend, this gives the clinical director little understanding of the real underlying problem. Money is a useful common denominator and helps to measure variation from a plan (or a budget) but the clinical director really needs to know *how* the workload of the directorate differs from what was expected.

Workload information

Many managers will be familiar with the dialogue set out in Figure 9.4. There are often very considerable quantities of information available within NHS trusts and the problem is often to decide what is relevant and what you need to manage. It is sometimes worth considering how we would approach the issue of measuring workload in a more reduced environment.

Measuring clinical work

Imagine, if you can, your appointment as administrator and manager of a small hospital in a rural part of the third world. Upon arrival you meet the existing manager, who is clearly due for retirement and who speaks only 'pidgin' English. Having walked around the place and seen the wards, you already know that the hospital treats quite a considerable number of in-patients and you ask him about this, as it is likely to be the area where the most money is being spent. 'Yes, yes 5000 last year' he tells you proudly. You begin to feel a bit more secure. Five thousand inpatients – that is quite a significant workload. In response to a question on what sort of patients, he again smiles broadly and says 'Some cut, some baby, some tummy, some car smash and some die'. Well it seems as if there is some surgery, some obstetrics, general medicine, accident and emergency and possibly ter-minal care. It seems unlikely that there is a gastroenterology department so you take this to be a short hand for more general medical problems. You feel you are beginning to get somewhere and ask him for a bit more detail about the cases treated in the previous year. He reaches into the desk drawer, pulls out a huge bundle of keys and proudly marches you down the corridor to a room marked '1997'. He swings open the door with a flourish and shows you shelves, heaving and groaning with case notes of every description. They are all in coloured files with symbols on the out-side and annotations in the local language. 'Everything you want to know here' he says. A week later, with the help of an assistant, you begin to make some sense of things. Each different doctor has a different colour code, so it is relatively simple to count the number of patients treated by each doc-tor. You know that the medical staff are very varied, ranging from keen European volunteers with a sense of vocation, working here for the experi-ence, through phlegmatic and cynical ex-pats who, for one reason or another, are unlikely to return to England, to the local man with private practice and family connections with the governing authority. Of course you know that just looking at the number of patients treated will not give you an indication of the relative burden being taken by the different doc-tors and their teams. You are going to need to know something about the type of patients, over and above some broad specialty categorization. ICD 10 is of course not used here and there is probably no one competent to code the record. However, each detailed and painstakingly completed record does have some diagnostic conclusion and this indicates either the major body area affected or the systemic disease. Your assistant suggests assigning each case to a chapter of the ICD as a first step. You agree and begin to think of one or two specific clusters in each chapter that you feel could be easily identified. For example, malaria, tuberculosis, road traffic accidents, malnutrition, etc.

At this stage you are about to invent DRGs, or some local variant!

NHS data

As it would be in a foreign country, so it is in an English NHS trust, but the information you want is available here and could be organized in a way that could be helpful to you. You need to understand the work that the directorate does and it is very likely that your first focus will be on inpatient work, which consumes up to 80% of the total resource of most clinical directorates in acute trusts. Because of this, since 1948, a variety of data collection systems has been put in place in the NHS and throughout the UK a uniform data set is collected. Your business manager, by bribing, threatening or otherwise coercing the information department ought to be able to get the information that you want into something like the format that you desire. A simple start would be to look at the workload of the department for the last year, acknowledging that there is occasionally a gap between the discharge of a patient and the creation of the full record and that you are safest looking at a period that finished two or three months previously.

You will want to look at the numbers of cases being treated by each consultant or clinical team, the length of time individual cases are in hospital and the average for groups of cases and understand something of the nature of the cases being undertaken. Of course you will know personally and from working with colleagues the sorts of cases they treat. 'I know John does complex fractures and Peter tends to do hernia repairs', for example. What is important is to get a comprehensive overview of the work being done and an understanding of the kinds of resources involved. A typical directorate is likely to deal with some 5000 or more cases in a year and the problem will be to try to analyse these cases. If you ask for a printout showing the diagnostic code and the operation code linked to each inpatient record you will face a huge mass of unsorted data. There are some 10 000 disease codes and 6000 operation codes and a very wide variety is likely to occur in any directorate.

Pareto and HRGs

There are two essential management tools which can help clinical directors understand and deal with the very considerable volume of information they face. The first is a general tool, the Pareto principle and the second is health service specific and is a classification system; DRGs, or in the UK, HRGs. The Pareto principle draws on distribution theory and normal distributions to suggest that around 80% of work derives from the 20% most common diagnoses. It reminds us that management analysis need not and should not be comprehensive, but needs to focus on the main issue. Rather than get lost in the complexities of the very occasional case we should try to understand the broad thrust of what the directorate is undertaking. Healthcare Resource Groups are described more fully elsewhere in this book but provide a basic, clinician friendly, analytic tool. A typical directorate is likely to see 80% of its case load expressed by between 20 and 50 HRGs.

What is important is not only that you as clinical director understand the workload of the directorate, but that your perceptions are validated and shared with the other stakeholders, particularly consultant colleagues. If you are going to suggest change based on your analysis you will need, at minimum, to have general agreement about the validity of the numerate and rational aspects of your proposal.

Managing change

Derek Pugh from Aston University[2] suggests that change needs to be managed consciously on three different levels. He designates these as the rational, the political and the professional. It is important that there are rational arguments for change and that these are discussed and debated and that there is agreement about a rational case. This in itself does not preclude the need to manage political and professional aspects of change and is therefore a necessary but not sufficient element of change management.

How should you tackle the issue of HRG analysis of workload within the directorate? Initially, you will need to ensure that the trust as a whole has access to good quality expertise about HRGs. There must be someone, either based within the trust or easily accessible to the trust, who really does understand the various versions of HRGs and understands how the software works and who can liaise with the National Casemix Office in the event of queries or issues. If that expertise is not available then the clinical director and business manager will need to convince the trust executive of the need to develop that resource as a first step towards management of workload.

Having ensured that the requisite specialist expertise is available, the next step would be, through one means or another, to obtain a standard analytic

Table 9.1:   An example of an analytic report for consultant A

HRG	Cases	Consultant A mean LoS	Standard deviation	Trust mean LoS
f32 colon and rectum procedures category 5	32	13.6	2.4	13.3
f33 colon and rectum procedures category 4	41	9.9	2.1	11.1
f84 appendix procedures category 3	51	4.1	1.1	3.6
f73 hernia procedures category 4	70	2.1	1.1	1.3
Etc.				

report of, say, one year's workload data, showing, perhaps, for each HRG a breakdown by consultant showing numbers of cases and mean length of stay, as well as standard deviation. An example is set out in Table 9.1.

The clinical director, business manager and HRG specialist would then need to work carefully through the entire analysis, trying to understand each line and compiling a list, to be investigated, of first-level reactions and particular concerns about the basic data.

Clinical coding

The assignment of an HRG category to an inpatient record depends mainly on the diagnosis and operation code. In some instances the existence of additional supplementary diagnoses is important to indicate relevant co-morbidities. Clinical directors will want to understand and think through each step between the patient discharge and the coding of the underlying cause for the hospital admission and the operations or interventions. There are some important conventions involved in coding to the standard of the ICD and, as with HRGs, it is important to establish that the hospital has a body of expertise and that it is available to support the directorate. In the end the only person who can authoritatively state the basic clinical diagnosis must be the consultant. The involvement of others in the process including junior medical staff and record and coding specialists needs, at minimum, to be quality assured. Clinical directors really carry the respons-ibility for all coded records that relate to their directorate and it is often salutary to begin to work through the variety of people involved. In some trusts the consultant staff see the assignation of the diagnosis as an important part of the teaching process and regard their quality control of the juniors' work as determining whether they have genuinely understood the clinical elements of each case. It is possible to have diagnostic coding checked by external benchmarking agencies who will review a variety of case notes and compare their results with local coders, but a simple regular routine review is probably at least as effective. It is important to remember that the coded aspects of the case are the only diagnostic information held on computers unless a local audit system is in place and that the true clinical richness of the patient needs to be properly recorded if this database is to, in any way, provide analysis of workload. A workload of 100 revision hip replacements per annum is very different to a workload of 100 primary hip replacements.

HRG review

Once the clinical director, business manager and local coding HRG specialist have 'cleaned up' the basic data and are satisfied that the HRG analysis of the directorate is broadly accurate, then the analysis could be introduced as a topic for discussion between the clinical director and the rest of the directorate staff on an individual or group basis. At this point it must be presented as a review of the basic information rather than making any attempt to draw conclusions from it. The aim is quite simply to gain agreement with consultant colleagues and other stakeholders within the directorate that the HRG analysis does properly represent the work being done. A colleague who said 'I do five of those in my theatre session every Tuesday and I would expect to see about 250 not 140!' may have a point and there may be miscoded cases lurking elsewhere. Alternatively he or she may have forgotten the cancelled sessions for holidays, working for the Royal College and other distractions. It sometimes helps, when looking at an HRG, to identify a particular patient who could be regarded as 'typical' of that HRG. Thus HRG 43 could be described as 'This is a group of the sort of case that Joe Bloggs represented'. Information systems specialists can help to identify modal patients in each HRG; that is those with the most common LoS and most typical diagnosis.

It may be that some HRGs contain considerable numbers of patients and, locally at least, are thought to have two or more quite distinct groups within them. There is no reason not to subdivide HRGs further if it makes local sense, although care should be taken not to move into very small groups. Similarly, a number of HRGs of quite small numbers may, locally at least, be seen as sensible if combined. What is important is to retain some 'mapping' back to the nationally agreed set of HRGs in order to be able to continue to make comparisons with other NHS organizations.

The value of HRG analysis is to provide a comparative framework. Having cleared up and agreed some local data sets you can begin to compare numbers and LoS with similar data from other organizations, either using data from the National Casemix Office or paying a commercial company to provide comparative data.

Clinical audit

Audit is a vital activity within a directorate and clinical directors must take responsibility for ensuring that proper audit is being conducted. In fact most clinical directors appoint an audit lead and leave it to them to organize the audit meetings. In some cases this works well, but in others the result is often a series of audit topics chosen for reasons of varying validity. The availability of a registrar, a complaint from someone, an article spotted in the *BMJ* or a request from the college can often drive local audit programmes. Whilst clinical audit is a unique activity in its own right, the management of an audit programme is not unique and finance, in particular, has dealt for 50 years at least, with the idea of applying a limited resource to a large task. Financial audit plans ensure that over a period, of say five years, they cover all financial systems and use a technique known as 'risk weighting' to put smaller amounts of resource into those areas of little potential risk and considerable resource into those areas where there are significant risks. The same kind of principle can be adopted within a directorate to plan a rolling programme of audit designed to cover all the work of the directorate over perhaps a five-year period and still allow some time for contingency and 'trouble shooting' audits. Those conditions which are rare and unusual, and yet where treatment is relatively stable and defined, are likely to be poor candidates for significant audit studies. On the other hand, those common procedures which have little 'clinical sexiness' may nevertheless be ideal candidates. The kind of framework that HRG analysis provides will support this kind of thinking and planning.

Treatment protocols

The role of the clinical director in developing and agreeing standards for clinical work is sometimes not fully acknowledged. There still exists, at least in some trusts, a convenient myth that audit is in some way disconnected from management and is about the professional practice of clinical medicine without consideration of resource. In the end this cannot be true since all choices about treatment have implications for the resources of directorate as a whole and the approach in many directorates has been to develop protocols to deal with the most frequent groups of patients. The debate still rages about the nomenclature; protocols, guidelines, standards and so on are often used interchangeably, but can sometimes be loaded terms. What is important is to acknowledge the uniqueness of each patient and the necessarily unique clinical response, whilst at the same time agreeing a local pattern of practice, variation from which will require justification.

A recent BAMM survey showed that some 90% of all clinical directorates are developing protocols and that these currently cover up to 25% of trust workload. The majority, 69%, are developing protocols which cover all aspects of a case; referral, treatment and discharge.

Whilst treatment protocols can, in theory at least, be developed entirely within the trust without reference to other practitioners, both referral and discharge protocols will need discussion and debate with other professionals, particularly GPs and colleagues in primary care. Of course it might be helpful to involve them in discussions on the treatment protocols as well, if only to help them gain a detailed understanding of what, typically, the directorate does for specific types of patients. More importantly however the discussion on referral protocols can smooth the whole patient episode, ensuring that there is an agreement on what tests and other work-up are already conducted before the patient reaches the hospital. Geriatricians and those with interests in the elderly have, for many years, practised working to discharge protocols to try to ensure appropriate collaboration with social services and other agencies. Acute specialties are now also beginning to develop protocols in this area. Developing protocols for specific HRGs means that the initial choice of patient groups is likely to be acknowledged as a homogeneous group of individuals and there will already be some data on variation in resource use, at least within the hospital.

Forecasting

Once there is a robust and commonly accepted HRG analysis of the directorate workload, perhaps drawn from a previous year's data, it provides an excellent framework for discussion on future patient numbers. It will quickly become apparent that treatment modalities and referral rates are relatively stable for a number of HRGs whilst others are demonstrating growth in numbers and in others, clinicians are known to be modifying treatment regimens or indeed applying new therapies. The ability of such a framework to focus debate and indicate areas where better information is required can materially support discussion with health authorities on shifts in casemix and resource use.

The above description suggests a somewhat reactive approach of trying to respond to change. A more proactive perspective is clearly possible; where those HRG groups which are either high in number or known to be high in resource use, can be aggressively reviewed to determine the potential for modifying treatment approaches or working with primary care practitioners to reduce the numbers requiring secondary care services.

Visioning

Few clinical directors are comfortable with the idea of developing a vision within the directorate and most find strategic planning difficult, particularly when the directorate is large and embraces a number of specialties, some of which are less familiar to them. Once again the use of the HRG analysis as a basic framework for discussion and debate can often be helpful. Using the Pareto principles and focusing on those 20 or 30 HRGs that bring with them 80% of the work of the directorate, it is possible to review each of these groups of patients in turn, asking questions such as 'What developments in treatment are we likely to see over five to ten years with these patients?', 'How are things changing for this sort of patient?', or even 'Will the prognosis for this kind of case improve – what is going to cause this improvement?'. Individual specialists and clinical teams may already be aware of new therapies and new technology, or those which are still being developed – the pharmaceutical compound still in the middle of the R&D programme, for example. Some early appreciation of the potential impact of these kinds of breakthroughs can give the clinical director valuable strategic understanding of the way the work of the directorate may change in the future. The closeness of clinicians to clinical development is one of their great strengths as clinical managers and the failure of the NHS to draw lessons from the past is very visible. It seems extremely clear that these kinds of debate and discussions were not held with the introduction of, for example, cimetidine to name but one example.

Decision-making

A clinical director armed with a deep understanding of the workload of the directorate, confident that those aspects of clinical work that can be systematized are being, and with some perspective on likely change both in the short term and the medium to long term, is well equipped to play a

corporate role within the organization as well as managing the directorate. It is of course imperative that the management system (that is the roles,
structures and groups which tackle key management processes such as
budgeting and planning) support and allow the clinical director to play a
full role. A description of appropriate management arrangements to involve clinical staff in the management of NHS trusts is outside the brief of
this chapter but much material and discussion can be found in Managing
Clinical Services.[3] What is important is that whatever system the clinical
director engages with, they are able to present rational arguments as well
as marshalling political and professional approaches to change.

Clinical directors in non-acute trusts

Much of the above is written around the clinical director of an acute trust.
The great advantage of the acute sector is that there are well established
data systems for inpatients. Clinical directors in mental health, learning
disability or community trusts face a very different challenge. Here again
the critical thing is to be able, in some way, to analyse the activity of the
directorate and break it up into constituent elements and begin to look at
groups and clusters of activity. The National Casemix Office has experi-
mental work on ambulatory groups and a number of developments in the
community field. Mental health and psychiatric disorders have also been
tackled and discussion with the National Casemix Office will identify
leading trusts in this area. The underlying principle is however the same.
The clinical director, supported by information from the NCMO or in any
other way needs to establish in conjunction with key stakeholders within
the directorate what are in general agreed to be similar groups of clients or
patients who 'evoke a similar clinical response and consume similar quantities of resource'. It is this grouping together of patients and treatment
episodes which is fundamental to the concept of HBGs and HRGs, which
allows and supports management processes.

References

1   British Association of Medical Managers (1997) *The Evolving Role of
    the Clinical Director*. BAMM, Manchester.
2   Pugh D (1978) Undertaking and managing organisational change.
    London Business School Journal 3(2): 29–34.
3   British Association of Medical Managers (1996) *Managing Clinical
    Services – principles into practice*. BAMM, BMA, IHSM and RCN.

10   Health benefit groups in NHS decision-making

ANDREW WALKER, KAREN JACK, SARA TWADDLE AND HARRY BURNS*

Introduction

Few would doubt that decision-making in the NHS is an art form rather than a science. A number of unavoidable factors make rational decision-making difficult, including the politically sensitive nature of the health service and the number of interest groups involved. Research attention has increasingly focused on ways in which decision-makers can be helped to work within these constraints. There is a general problem with the lack of an evidence base which can be used to make judgements; there is also a more specific problem about the lack of a framework for discussions between purchasers, providers, and other stakeholders regarding the development of health services. The evidence base is being slowly assembled via the NHS Centre for Reviews and Dissemination, Effective Health Care Bulletins and the NHS Research and Development programme. Some progress has been made with standardizing data for use in discussions, such as HRGs, as a means of casemix adjustment. This chapter discusses HBGs/HRG matrices, which seek to summarize existing information about a health service as a basis for discussions and decisions.

Health Benefit Groups have been developed by the NCMO of the NHS Executive as a framework for NHS decision-makers. There are two separate concepts: first, there is the HBG itself, which is intended to be an iso-need grouping of people. If cancer stage is a good predictor of prognosis then different cancer stages might form different HBGs at the treatment stage, for example. The second element of the approach is to set these HBGs within a series of pre-defined tables that bring together epidemiological, health service activity and finance data. Different sets of tables cover different disease groups (such as the common cancers) as well as client groups (such as female sexual health). Ultimately, it is intended to include outcomes and structure/process data in the tables (see Appendix in Chapter 1). For simplicity, we will continue to refer to both the HBG groupings and the table as HBGs.

*At the time of the project all of the authors were employed by Greater Glasgow Health Board.

However, assembling and interpreting data are potentially costly activities in terms of staff time and (possibly) additional data collection. How can we be sure that this time is being put to its most effective use? To address this question, this chapter seeks to identify some of the potential benefits and costs of HBGs. We have drawn on the experience of Greater Glasgow Health Board (GGHB) as the pilot site for sets of matrices covering breast, lung and colorectal cancer between October 1996 and June 1997. This has allowed us to start to identify the circumstances under which HBGs are most likely to be cost-effective.

The anatomy of an HBG matrix

To understand what HBGs might achieve, and some of the potential problems in practice, this section presents a brief description of a set of matrices. Typically, there are five matrices in a set, covering:

1 primary prevention
2 diagnosis
3 treatment
4 follow-up, and
5 a summary sheet showing totals from the other four sheets.

The vertical axis of each table contains the HBGs, defined as groups of people with broadly similar needs. In the case of cancer, pathological staging might be an example. On the horizontal axis, the first column shows the number of people falling into the HBG; subsequent columns cover the health services that they might receive. At present, only some of these columns can be specified in terms of an HRG code (or codes). As HRG development progresses more columns will be identified as HRGs and ultimately this should be possible for all of them.

A selection of the data from the set of matrices on colorectal cancer is shown in Table 10.1 as an example. Matrix 1 shows the epidemiological risk factors associated with the disease with estimates of the numbers of people in the GGHB population thought to be at increased risk. Matrix 2 shows the diagnostic tests for the various types of presentation. Matrix 3 shows the primary treatment of colorectal cancer using Dukes' staging as the basis for HBGs. These are aggregated together in the summary matrix but in this instance no information was available on the needs for supportive/palliative care or services provided, so only the first three matrices were used.

Table 10.1: Summary sheet for colorectal cancer: matrices

Summary matrix

	Promotion and primary prevention	Investigation and diagnosis	Initial care	Continuing care	TOTAL
At risk	£152 381				
Presentation		£38 097	£339 200		
Confirmed disease			£3 438 609		
Continuing disease states				£?	
Total					£3 968 287

Matrix 1: Primary and secondary prevention of disease

	Prevalence	Health promotion	FOB	Screening Endoscopic	Genetic	Special support	TOTAL
Whole population	916 600	£50 000					
Low risk							
Age 50+	282 514						
High-fat, low-fibre diet	401 684	£50 000					
Positive family history	28 251						
Ulcerative colitis	1467						
Ureterosigmoidostomy							
High risk							
Previous history of CRC	3042			£45 433			
HNPCC	170			£6949			
FAP	26						
Total		£100 000	£0	£52 381	£0	£0	£152 381

HNPCC Hereditary non-polyposis carcinoma colon
FAP Familial adenosis polyposi
FOB Faecal occult blood

Table 10.1: Continued

Matrix 2: Diagnosis of disease

	Prevalence	Examn. bloods, FOB	Endoscopy	Emergency laparotomy	Ultrasound	CT	Special support	TOTAL
Asymptomatic/ screened detected	27	£3360	£7082	£0	£853	£2073	£0	£0
Symptomatic local	334	£42 339	£89 235	£0	£8059	£19 591	£0	
Pain	134							
Mass	100							
Rectal bleeding	110							
Change bowel habit	234							
Obstruction	33							
Perforation	20							
Generalized								
Weight loss	200							
Vomiting	150							
Anaemia	100							
Emergency admission	170	£10 753	£22 663	£339 200	£1364	£3317	£0	£377 466
Total	530	£56 451	£118 980	£339 200	£10 276	£24 981	£0	

Matrix 3: Treatment of diagnosed disease

	Prevalence	Surgery Ops on colon	Ops on rectum	Liver resection	Chemotherapy Group 1	Group 2	Group 3	Group 4	Radiotherapy Simple palliative	Complex	Special support
Dukes A	53	£88 067	£67 187	£0	£0	£0	£0	£0	£0	£0	£10 600
Dukes B	159	£330 251	£251 951	£0	£0	£0	£0	£0	£0	£0	£31 800
Dukes C	186	£385 293	£293 943	£0	£571 665	£364 229	£169 733	£0	£62 662	£0	£37 100
Dukes D	133	£206 407	£157 470	£33 125	£0	£104 066	£121 238	£0	£125 324	£0	£26 500
Total	530	£1 010 017	£770 551	£33 125	£571 665	£468 295	£290 970	£0	£187 986	£0	£106 000

Chemotherapy groups relate to complexity of drug regime (1 = simplest, 4 = most complex)

The potential of HBG matrices

To plan services on the basis of evidence is very demanding of information about deficiencies in the current service, options for remedying these deficiencies and the marginal costs and benefits of implementing these options. Health Benefit Groups offer a framework for such discussions by describing the current service using the best available data (deficient as this might be) and presenting the opportunity for examining the consequences of changes in the volume and nature of work in terms of activity and costs. By summarizing the data in a format that can be analysed on a simple computer spreadsheet, HBGs offer managers the scope to understand local health services in detail.

This information could be used to look at the balance of spending across a range of services or to launch a more detailed scrutiny of a single service. It has the advantage of summarizing data that might fall under a number of different administrative headings, including those outside of the NHS.

To illustrate the range of potential applications, it is possible to assemble a number of ideas under two different headings. The first of these is 'Understanding Demand' and includes six potential applications.

1 Examine the implications of purchasing the whole programme of care for a condition.
2 Understand the implications of changing the balance of expenditure for different treatments.
3 Record baseline figures for measurement of change over time.
4 Assess need for services locally.
5 Understand typical health care needs of diseases.
6 Contribute to weighting factors for groups, such as the elderly, and to allow for socio-economic factors.

Four further applications are listed under the heading 'Focus Resource Use'.

1 Inform decisions on distribution of resources and adjustments to services provided.
2 Assist resource allocation changes and improve interfaces between purchasers and providers.
3 Indicate workload and cost implications of moving activity, for example from secondary to primary, or from hospital to long-stay facilities.
4 Help focus resources to meet Health of the Nation targets.

This suggests that the main use of HBGs would be by commissioners/planners of health services, whether they be at a national, regional, district or GP level. Providers may also find the information valuable, particularly in terms of performance comparisons, but the remainder of this chapter assumes that the main users will be district health authorities or GP commissioners. We return to this issue in the discussion. The next section considers some of the problems with HBGs before the final section attempts to identify their most valuable role.

Barriers to realizing the potential of HBGs

So far we have described HBGs and outlined their potential applications. However, pilot studies have also identified a number of issues relating to the matrices. These include:

- ability to complete matrices from existing data sources and the quality of the data obtainable from those sources
- valuation of resource use
- choice of HBGs
- inclusion of outcome measures.

This section considers these in turn, together with proposed solutions to these problems.

Ability to complete matrices from existing data sources

The project team had to make decisions at the outset regarding the scope of the exercise. For example, should the matrices summarize the experience of a cohort of patients over time, or should they be a 'snapshot' for a single year with patients at a number of different stages of the disease (and treatment) process? Similarly, should they be completed at a population level or by each provider unit? Finally, should the matrices include costs incurred outside of the NHS, including voluntary or charitable bodies and informal carers? As the project was based in a commissioning agency, it was decided to use a 'snapshot' population perspective on resource use that had implications for the budget of the local purchaser. Even these apparently straightforward decisions had implications for the use of the matrices, as demonstrated in later sections.

The main problem encountered after this was with existing data sources. The colorectal cancer matrices shown drew heavily upon the previous experience of two members of the research team. Where this in-depth knowledge was not available, the matrices were harder to complete. For example, in the matrix for breast cancer treatment only 21 of the

56 cells could be completed or just over one-third of the potentially relevant information.

Even to achieve this level required considerable supplementation of existing data sources. The number of operations with a particular diagnostic code can be calculated from these sources but there are no data on the cancer stage. Indeed, in the cancer matrices *none* of the HBG classifications are yet currently collected under routine data collection, hence the pilot study also used audit data (both local and national) to estimate the proportions of activity of particular types relating to different HBGs. These data were supplied by the Scottish Cancer Therapy Network and by GGHB. Audit staff responded to *ad hoc* requests, a facility that will not be available in all areas or for all subjects. Neither audit project was designed with this type of exercise in mind and some of the data sets used represent practice as it was five years ago. To complete the matrices some assumptions were made, such as the applicability of cancer staging distributions found in a national audit several years ago to current activity in Glasgow. As a simple validity check, local clinicians working in the relevant fields were asked for their comments on the figures; in general, the assumptions made were thought to be reasonable. However, audit data tend to be collected through acute hospitals and will thus focus on this aspect of the health service to the exclusion of the community and primary care services.

One solution to this problem would be to re-design the routine NHS data collection systems so that they collected more of the data required, such as the stage of different cancers at diagnosis. However, this would add to the cost of data collection and would slow the collection of data that are gathered for other purposes – for example, awaiting full cancer staging information may involve a delay in submitting discharge information of several weeks. As GP data systems improve it may be possible to make more use of them as a source at some stage in the future: at present there are problems with the completeness of these data and with interrogating the databases. This source may prove particularly useful where GPs provide a substantial proportion of the care, such as in diabetes or asthma.

Another solution would be to use other *ad hoc* data sources, such as reviewing the hospital case notes and GP records of patients identified through the Cancer Registry. Again, this would add to the cost of the exercise, particularly if a number of matrices were being completed; with management cost restrictions, this seems unlikely. In any case, such sources are not designed for this purpose and would still require supplementation from other sources. Prospective data collection would suffer from similar problems.

A third option would be to simplify future versions of the matrices and thus reduce the number of cells to be completed. There are problems with such an approach: ideally, the specification of the matrices would stem from a careful identification of the potential role of the matrices in decision-making. On the other hand, the Glasgow pilot identified some areas where the information appeared redundant or very difficult to interpret: the format of the matrix on the follow-up to initial therapy requires considerable revision, for example. This suggests that there is scope to modify the first attempt at the matrices without loss of useful detail.

Valuation of resource use

In Glasgow, detailed HRG costs are only slowly becoming available, hence the matrices were completed on the basis of price tariffs for GP fundholders and of average specialty costs from routine financial returns. Although NHS Executive guidance to trusts demands that price tariffs be set equal to costs, the inevitable subjectivity inherent in allocating overhead costs and the costs of resources used by a number of services cast some doubt on whether these prices truly reflect the value of resources used in a procedure. HRG costs will be helpful in this respect but are not routinely available for all trusts at present. The matrices must thus be interpreted with caution.

The use of average costs (or prices) to value resources consumed also creates problems for decision-making 'at the margin'. Even if decision-makers were to make detailed decisions about purchasing a few more or a few less of a particular procedure they would wish to know the additional resources involved: these may not equal the average cost. If marginal cost is less than average cost then the matrices as presently calculated will tend to overstate the savings of reducing activity and overstate the costs of expanding services.

One solution would be to concentrate on activity data in the matrices, only estimating additional costs when a change in the service is being considered. This may force decision makers to consider which types of resources are the most valuable in the sense of being scarce or causing 'bottlenecks' at present. Another possibility would be to educate users of the matrices as to the difference between average and marginal cost: a simple rule of thumb (marginal cost equals a given percentage of average cost) could be used to guide decisions. Further refining of average costs will be of no value in this respect.

Choice of HBGs

As noted above, the HBGs are the iso-need groups represented as the rows of the matrices. One problem noted above is that none of these feature in routine resource collection systems. However, the basis on which the HBGs are chosen is also unclear. In Matrix 1 (Table 10.1, page 113) the basis appears to reflect increased relative risk of being diagnosed with the disease, but it is not clear what evidence is required to support inclusion in the matrices. In Matrix 2 the choice of symptoms creates extreme difficulties for data collection, especially when the symptoms are so common. In Matrix 3, cancer stage is one basis for looking at iso-need groups, but others could be operations that are palliative and curative or colonic and rectal tumours.

One way to clarify these issues would be to make clear the basis upon which each classification had been chosen, even if this involves comparatively arbitrary decisions such as a cut-off point in terms of relative risk for inclusion in Matrix 1.

Inclusion of outcomes

Decisions are commonly based on a range of factors, among which the implications for health and resource use are prominent. In the pilot project the matrices only included costs. Outcomes are multi-dimensional and are rarely collected routinely. To illustrate, consider what data would be required to judge the outcomes of cancer services. The first stage is to determine what each element of the service is trying to achieve and then to identify a reliable and valid indicator to measure performance. A simple framework, which is not intended to be definitive, is set out in Table 10.2.

As the final column illustrates, gathering a comprehensive range of outcome measures is itself a costly activity. In addition, a number of potentially confounding variables would have to be collected so that variations in outcomes over time or as a cross-section could be interpreted. Finally, long-term outcomes (such as survival rates at five years following diagnosis) may not be available until some time after the activity that is intended to affect it. Any given matrix may thus compare 1998 activity with the results of the services available in 1993.

From the above it is clear that outcomes can be collected and included in the matrices, but the cost may be considerable and may delay production of the matrices. As an alternative, evidence-based guidelines for the management of cancers have been developed which, if adhered to, are expected to produce the best outcomes that can be achieved. The task of management would then be to monitor adherence to these guidelines. Health Benefit Groups can provide some assistance, but only to the extent that the recommended actions from the guidelines will show in routine activity statistics. For example, if it were recommended that all stage C colon cancers undergoing surgery should receive chemotherapy, then HBGs could assist in monitoring adherence. On the other hand, they could not

Table 10.2:   Multiple outcomes for a cancer matrix

Matrix	Dimensions of outcome	Possible data sources
1 Prevention	i) Cancers prevented	Cancer Registry, no extra cost
	ii) Public knowledge about cancer	Surveys already carried out, little extra cost
	iii) Changes in risky behaviour	Surveys already carried out, little extra cost
	iv) Asymptomatic cancers detected at early stage	Could not be identified from Cancer Registry, further data collection required
	v) Reassurance (especially for genetic high-risk patients)	Survey methods possible, no routine data collected, extra cost
2 Diagnosis	i) Accurate diagnosis (high sensitivity and specificity)	Requires follow-up of patients to determine cancers missed, further data collection, extra cost
	ii) Speed of diagnosis	Sampling approach possible, further data collection, extra cost
	iii) Anxiety/injury from diagnostic investigation	Survey methods possible, no routine data collected, extra cost
3 Treatment	i) Survival after diagnosis	Available from Cancer Registry but not classified into HBGs, further data collection required, extra cost
	ii) Physical and mental health status	Survey methods possible, no routine data collected, extra cost
	iii) Impact on carer	Survey methods possible, no routine data collected, extra cost
4 Follow-up	As above plus i) Anxiety/depression	Survey methods possible, no routine data collected, extra cost
	ii) Dignity/autonomy in terminal care	Survey methods possible, no routine data collected, extra cost
	iii) Symptom control	Survey methods possible, no routine data collected, extra cost

show whether the cancer had been adequately staged or whether the surgeon had adhered to best practice in resecting the cancer.

Applications of HBG matrices

The previous section discussed ways to tackle some of the practical difficulties with completing HBGs: most could be addressed, albeit at a cost. What implications do these issues have for the use of HBG matrices in NHS decision-making? From the list of potential applications listed above, which are most likely to demonstrate the value of the approach?

Applications with current data sources

The matrices are not a panacea. In the format used in the pilot for colorectal cancer, they do not incorporate outcome and process measures and therefore do not address important questions such as comparisons between providers in terms of resource use and outcome, comparisons between clinicians in terms of outcome (to address issues about specialization of treatment) or about the appropriate role of primary care teams in disease management. Of course, less aggregated formats with outcome and process indicators could be used but involve extra complexity and cost to complete and interpret.

The next point to consider is to whom the matrices might be of use. From the Glasgow pilot study of cancer, reactions were mixed. Hospital clinicians gave the clearest set of responses: while they welcomed attempts to describe their service, especially if they were designed to correspond with evidence-based guidelines, none felt that the current matrices would be of use in guiding their day-to-day practice. One concern was that the matrices took no account of comorbidity. Hospital managers were generally receptive to the information, although there was concern that the information presented in the matrices was far more detailed than that used for discussions about contracts with purchasers.

Purchasers also felt that the information would be interesting, but there was less consensus about their usefulness: some were interested in disaggregating block contracts, whereas others felt that so long as designated treatment specialists were managing patients then purchasers could concentrate on other areas. Purchasers generally did not want to become involved in detailed clinical decision-making. However, one purchaser commented that HBGs could become much more important if HRGs were the routine contract currency.

General practitioners also welcomed the attempt to assemble information although they were less clear about specific applications: it should be noted that cancer services may not be the best example to demonstrate the potential value of HBGs in primary care. However, it was felt that GPs would be interested in aspects of the matrices such as finding out how many patients referred with a cough were diagnosed as having lung cancer.

For each of the three groups, the potential applications could have been achieved by *ad hoc* means: for example, GPs were interested to know how many referrals for a particular indication resulted in a diagnosis of cancer. This could be addressed by a literature review or analysis of outpatient statistics without requiring a full set of HBG matrices.

Given some of the difficult issues described above, it seems likely that the first uses of HBG matrices will be at a summary level. For example, they might allow comparisons of the *total* spent on preventing colorectal cancer versus the *total* spent on treating symptomatic disease. This, in itself, will move the debate forward: for instance, one purchaser may compare the proportion of total spend on preventative services with the same figure in a neighbouring area, and then explore the reasons for major differences.

However, such comparisons are limited without evidence on the outcomes of spending for each type of service. In addition, the method of completing the matrices needs to be standardized. In the Glasgow pilot study of cancer matrices a number of *ad hoc* judgements were made about the validity of activity data of different vintages, the apportionment of totals between rows and columns and the valuation of resource use. For example, if the total number of operations for a particular diagnosis is known, and it is assumed that the staging distribution for cancer is as for Scotland as a whole then we can estimate activity by HBG for Glasgow. However, this is only an indirect estimate that may mask important variations between hospitals in Glasgow and variations over time. Local judgements will inevitably vary, producing differences between neighbouring services that are spurious (or masking genuine differences). The complexity of the exercise with incomplete data means that definitive rules would be difficult to draw up, although it may be possible to agree some guidelines. For example, this could help with the handling of data where the HBG is unknown e.g. an operation for unstaged colon cancer in Matrix 3, Table 10.1. In the future, when detailed clinical data are accessible (especially for GP systems), the rules for extraction and application will be easier.

Would better quality data help?

The single biggest step forward would be to include outcomes information in the matrices (as detailed in the Appendix in Chapter 1). However, as the section above describes, capturing this would be complex and costly. Without this information the matrices focus on activity and cost alone, encouraging managers to focus on what is easy to measure rather than what matters. This is not to say that as they stand the exercise has no value: it serves to facilitate dialogue between purchasers and providers and with GPs and others outside of the NHS. The quality of this dialogue would be greatly improved by the inclusion of outcomes and the costs of collecting these data should be considered at an early stage. There are also important issues about the outcome scale chosen, the numbers needed in a particular cell of a matrix to allow comparisons showing statistical significance, and so on.

More generally, better quality data or more comprehensive data sources would help but there may still be a problem if decision-making is at a cruder, more aggregated level than HBGs assume. In many areas of the country, because of the lack of data and systematic tools to handle it purchasing still uses modified versions of block contracts. Where purchasers take decisions about specific services these tend to be reactive, e.g. in response to a request from a trust for extra funding for a new drug.

In part, this may be due to the same lack of detailed data that creates problems for the completion of the matrices in the first place. However, this also reflects the time pressures faced by purchasers, limiting their ability to enter into detailed discussions about changes to clinical services. The matrices could form the basis of a regular round of reviews, possibly with commissioning agencies tackling two or three subjects each year. In this scenario, the matrices would not have to be completed for all topics every year: if the purchasers have decided that cardiovascular disease will be this year's priority then only the most relevant HBG matrices would be completed. This would also give greater prominence to hypothesis-driven data collection, focusing on the issues within a broad topic that are of specific local interest. While this would increase the relevance of the exercise to purchasers, any tailoring of the matrices would restrict comparisons between purchasers. This tension between allowing local purchasers to adapt the framework as they choose to meet local circumstances on the one hand, and the need for a clearly defined methodology that will allow comparisons between purchasers on the other hand, is a tension within the matrices that has not yet been completely resolved.

The experience of economists with programme budgeting, a comparable technique aimed at summarizing data to inform decisions about change, seems to bear this out. While the tables on current activity were thought to be useful descriptions of the current situation, using them to identify change proved more difficult. One problem was the reluctance of people involved to provide a service to identify ways to reduce that service, even if the savings were 'ring-fenced'. Another difficulty was the divergence between average costs and marginal costs to value resource use referred to above.

Summary and conclusion

This chapter describes the concept of the HBG and the matrices within which they can be used. Through examples from the pilot project in Glasgow, the potential of the matrices has been demonstrated as well as some of the difficulties with assembling the data and using the tables. The matrices have the greatest potential to assist as a framework for discussion and a means of prompting questions for further investigation. At present the quality of the data may restrict the application of the matrices beyond these roles. In particular, a standardized methodology for completing the matrices will be required before meaningful comparisons can be made between different purchasers in terms of their allocation of spending.

Acknowledgements

Particular thanks are due to Brian Merriman at the NCMO, as well as to Hugh Sanderson, Raju George and Sam Raymond. The following also assisted with helpful comments: Professor WD George, Dr N Reed, Professor T Habeshaw, Dr N O'Rourke, Dr R Jones, Professor T Cooke, Mr J Anderson, Dr I Colqhoune, Dr M Soukop, Dr D McIntyre, Dr R Milroy, Dr JC Ferguson, Dr R McKee, Dr R Davidson, Dr A Renwick and Dr E Mallon. Data were provided by Paul Stroner (Scottish Cancer Therapy Network), Eileen Kesson and Professor Charles Gillis. Despite the number of people involved in this project, we take full responsibility for all of the views and figures in this report.

Glossary and abbreviations

THE following list of definitions and abbreviations may be useful for readers of the casemix literature to help understand some of the materials.

casemix
The mix of types of patients or treatment episodes.

casemix classification
Classification of people or treatment episodes into groups, using characteristics associated with the condition, treatment or outcome that can be used to predict need, resource use or outcome.

cc
Complications and comorbidities.

CMG
Casemix group.

CMDS
Contract minimum data set.

complexity (casemix)
A measure of the complexity of activity or patients, in comparison to a standard population.

condition
Any health-related attribute of a patient.

DRG
Diagnosis Related Group.

efficiency (casemix)
A comparison of the actual cost/resource use for a group of patients to the expected cost/resource use, based on a standard cost/resource per HRG/DRG.

ECR
Extra-contractual referral.

FCE
Finished consultant episode. The period of time that one hospital inpatient spends under the care and responsibility of one consultant. There may be more than one FCE within a hospital stay.

GPFH   General practitioner fundholder.

HBG   Health Benefit Group. Groupings of people with similar conditions and similar expected outcomes.

HES   Hospital Episode Statistics. The English national data set for hospital inpatients.

HIPE   Hospital Inpatient Enquiry.

homogeneous   Uniformity within a casemix group.

HRG   Healthcare Resource Group. Groupings of treatment episodes which are similar in resource use and clinical response.

ICD   International Classification of Diseases. Internationally defined classification of disease; managed by the World Health Organization.

ICD 10   International Classification of Diseases. Tenth Revision.

ICD 9   International Classification of Diseases. Ninth Revision.

intervention   Clinical activity provided to manage the condition of a patient.

iso   Similar.

iso-resource   Similar in resource use.

length of stay (LoS) Duration of the finished consultant episode (FCE).

MDC   Major Diagnostic Category.

mean   The arithmetic average.

median   The value of the observation or case which is ranked exactly half way between the maximum and minimum values.

MDS	Minimum data set.
mode	The most frequent observation or case.
NCMO	National Casemix Office. Branch G of the Information Management Group of the NHS Executive, England.
Non-operative procedure (non-OR)	A procedure which is considered to be so minor that it does not affect the resources used within the FCE.
OPCS	Office of Population Censuses and Surveys (now the Office of National Statistics).
outcome	The change in condition of a patient or population resulting from intervention or treatment.
outlier	Any observation or case which is substantially higher or lower than the average. Normally identified by a statistical test; e.g. an episode with a length of stay greater than or equal to a specific trim point value.
PMC	Patient Management Category.
treatment	One or more clinical activities needed to determine or change the condition of a patient or population.
TPP	Total purchasing pilot.
trim point	Calculated using a statistical formula. The value above or below which an observation or case is determined to be substantially different to the main population.
trimming	A method of reducing the skewing of the mean length of stay by identifying and excluding outlier data.

Bibliography

THERE is a wide literature in casemix methods and applications which has grown up over the last 20 years. Much of this is focused on DRGs, and specifically derived from the USA where experience of developing and using casemix has been longer, and more intensive than anywhere else.

The key references from the USA include:

Fetter RB, Shin Y, Freeman JL *et al.* (1980) Casemix Definition by Diagnosis Related Groups. *Medical Care.* **18(Suppl.):** 1–53.

This is the definitive article describing the development and structure of DRGs.

Hornbrook MC (1983) Hospital Casemix: Its definition, measurement and use. *Medical Care Review.* **39:** 1–43.

An important review of the concepts and issues surrounding the construction of casemix measures.

Gonella JS, Hornbrook MC and Louis DZ (1984) Staging of Disease: a casemix measurement. *JAMA* **241:** 637–44.

Horn SD and Sharkey PD (1983) Severity of Illness to Predict Patient Resource Use within DRGs. *Inquiry* **20:** 314–21.

Young WW, Swinkola RB and Zorn DM (1982) The Measurement of Hospital Casemix. *Medical Care* **20:** 501–12.

These are descriptions of alternative models of casemix.

In Europe, Canada and Australia there has been an increasing amount of activity and writing in the last ten years. Important reviews of the developments in various countries are to be found in:

Casas M and Wiley MM (eds) (1993) *Diagnosis Related Groups in Europe.* Springer-Verlag, Berlin.

Kimberly JR and de Pourville G (1993) The Migration of Managerial Innovation. *Diagnosis Related Groups and Health care Administration in Western Europe.* Jossey Bass, San Francisco.

There have been annual Casemix Conferences in Europe and in Australia for more than ten years. The proceedings are of variable availability but contain a wide range of descriptions of work in progress and applications of casemix methods in Europe and Australia. Papers on casemix are also occasionally given at more general Informatics Conferences, such as MIE.

UK

Useful reviews of the history of DRGs and use of casemix in England are contained in:

Newman T and Jenkins L (1991) *DRG Experience in England 1981–1991*. CASPE Research, London.

Bardsley M, Coles JM and Jenkins L (eds) (1989) *DRGs and Health Care: The management of casemix* (2nd edn). King Edward's Hospital Fund, London.

A number of documents and case studies are available as Occasional Papers from the National Casemix Office. These describe developments and applications of casemix methods, including the relevant Executive letters relating to the use of HRGs for costing. Details are available from the National Casemix Office, Highcroft, Romsey Road, Winchester, Hants, England SO22 5DH.

Index